Communication Disorders in Childhood Cancer

BRUCE E MURDOCH

Department of Speech Pathology and Audiology
The University of Queensland, Brisbane.

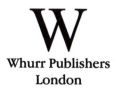

Whurr Publishers
London

© 1999 Whurr Publishers Ltd

First published 1999
by Whurr Publishers Ltd
19b Compton Terrace
London N1 2UN
England

British Library Cataloguing in Publication Data
A catalogue record for this book is available from the British Library.

ISBN 1 86156 115 6

Printed and bound in the UK by Athenaeum Press Ltd, Gateshead, Tyne & Wear

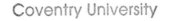

Contents

Preface

The survival rates of children treated for various neoplastic conditions such as brain tumours and acute lymphoblastic leukaemia have shown a dramatic improvement during the past three decades. Unfortunately it is now being recognized that treatments applied to these conditions, such as radiotherapy and chemotherapy, may have some long-term adverse effects on brain structure and function leading to the development of a number of negative sequelae. These sequelae include cognitive deficits as well as speech and language disorders. Consequently in recent years, an increasing number of children displaying communication deficits as a consequence of treatment for childhood cancer have begun to appear in the caseloads of speech pathologists and other health professionals. Further, the recognition that treatments for childhood cancer can be associated with a number of long-term negative outcomes has lead in recent years to a shift in the emphasis of research to include, in addition to improvement in survival rates, investigation of ways of improving the quality of life of survivors of childhood cancer.

During the past decade a group of researchers at the University of Queensland has undertaken a series of studies into the nature of speech and language disorders occurring in children treated for brain tumours and acute lymphoblastic leukaemia (ALL). These studies represent the most comprehensive reports of communication deficits in this population to date and have provided a platform for future research into speech and language problems occurring as an outcome of treatments such as radiotherapy and chemotherapy. The majority of these studies have been published as papers in *Aphasiology — An International Interdisciplinary Journal*. The permission of Taylor & Francis Ltd to reproduce some of the material contained in these papers in the present book is gratefully acknowledged.

The aim of the present book is to provide a synopsis of the research conducted at the University of Queensland over the past 10 years into communication impairments associated with childhood cancers. Its aim is to inform speech pathologists and other health professionals of the need to monitor the communication abilities of children treated for neoplastic conditions with a view to implementing appropriate treatment strategies where necessary. It is also intended that the book act as a stimulus for further research into the communication impairments experienced by children treated for cancer.

Bruce E Murdoch

List of contributors

Deborah L Boon (née Buttsworth) PhD Senior Speech Pathologist, Queensland Society for Crippled Children, Brisbane

Susan K Horton BAppSci (Speech Pathology) Lecturer in Speech Pathology, Department of Speech Pathology & Audiology, The University of Queensland

Lisa J Hudson PhD Senior Speech Pathologist, Toowoomba Base Hospital, Toowoomba, Queensland

Bruce E Murdoch PhD Professor and Head of Department, Department of Speech Pathology & Audiology, The University of Queensland

Chapter 1
Major childhood cancers: leukaemia and brain tumours

BRUCE E MURDOCH, DEBORAH L BOON AND
LISA J HUDSON

Introduction

The long-term quality of life experienced by survivors of paediatric cancer is an issue receiving increasing attention from allied health professionals. Of the paediatric malignancies, acute leukaemias are the most common (Parkin et al., 1988). Brain and spinal tumours are the second most common childhood cancer in the developed countries of North America, Europe and Australasia, with cited incidences ranging from 20 to 35 cases per million children (De Nully Brown et al., 1987; Parkin et al., 1988; Lannering et al., 1990; McWhirter and Petroeschevsky, 1990). In particular, tumours located in the posterior cranial fossa (i.e. infratentorial tumours involving the cerebellum, fourth ventricle and/or brainstem) occur more commonly in childhood than supratentorial neoplasms, accounting for up to 70% of all paediatric intracranial tumours (Hooper, 1975; Farwell et al., 1977; Gjerris, 1978; Segall et al., 1985; Kadota et al., 1989; Russell and Rubinstein, 1989).

Recent decades have seen developments in the treatment of paediatric cancer that have resulted in marked improvements in the five-year survival rates of children treated for neoplastic conditions. Although almost always rapidly fatal four decades ago (Southam et al., 1951; Tivey, 1952), the five-year survival rate of children treated for paediatric leukaemia in the 1990s has risen to 72.8% (Boring et al., 1991), with some survival rates reported to be as high as 80% (Cousens et al., 1990). Similarly, the survival rates for children diagnosed with brain and nervous system tumours have also shown dramatic improvement, with figures from the USA indicating improvement from 35% during the period 1960–1963 to 59% survival during the period 1981–1986 (Boring et al., 1991). Although indisputably saving the lives of children with neoplastic conditions, the treatments applied to these disorders, however, have been reported to induce structural and functional changes in the brain leading to the development of certain adverse long-term consequences which include, among others, speech and language deficits (Jackel et al., 1990; Hudson and Murdoch, 1992; Buttsworth et al., 1993). Consequently, the improvement in survival rates of children diagnosed with cancer has lead to allied health professionals, including speech/language pathologists, being required to provide rehabilitation and support services to an increasing number of paediatric cancer patients, with attention now focused on improving the quality of life of the survivors of childhood leukaemia and brain tumours.

The present chapter reviews the major types of paediatric cancers with regard to their epidemiology, diagnosis, aetiology, types, symptomatology, medical course and prognosis, with emphasis given to acute lymphoblastic leukaemia (ALL) and posterior cranial fossa tumours. The medical treatments applied to each of these latter conditions are also described. The effects of these treatments on brain structure and function are discussed in detail in Chapter 2.

Paediatric leukaemia

General features and epidemiology

Leukaemia is a progressive, malignant disease of the blood-forming organs, marked by distorted proliferation and development of leucocytes and their precursors in the blood and bone marrow. The most common form of leukaemia, ALL is associated with hyperplasia and overactivity of the lymphoid tissue. Most of the affected person's leucocytes in this condition are lymphocytes or lymphoblasts. Although ALL is a disease of children and adults, it predominantly affects children, with an initial peak incidence of the disease occurring between three and five years of age. Neglia and Robison (1988) pointed out that this peak does not occur uniformly throughout the world, and is not present in Africa and various developing nations (Edington and Hendrikse, 1973; Ansel and Nabemezi, 1974; Davies, 1985). The incidence of ALL decreases after five years of age, and drops sharply between the ages of 10 and 14 years (Madan-Swain and Brown, 1991). The incidence of ALL is higher in males than in females (Koocher and O'Malley, 1981) and, although the exact figures vary with the particular type, this sex pattern is consistent across geographical boundaries and racial groups (Neglia and Robison, 1988). One survey in the USA found that, for children under 15 years of age, the annual incidence of ALL among males was 22.3 per million, whereas for females it was 15.7 per million (Young and Miller, 1975).

As indicated earlier, although in past years ALL was almost invariably a fatal condition, improvements in survival times have occurred as a result of the development and introduction of more effective treatments since the beneficial effects of drug therapy were first described by Farber et al. (1948). In the 1960s, the chance of surviving five years after a diagnosis of ALL was 4% (Boring et al., 1991), and continued to improve so that, by the end of the 1970s, therapy for childhood ALL had become so effective that at least 50% of patients could expect to achieve long-term disease-free remission (Holland and Glidewell, 1972; Jacquillat et al., 1973; Till et al., 1973; Aur et al., 1978a; Crosley et al., 1978; Miller, 1980a, b; McCalla, 1985). Meadows et al. (1980) predicted that, by the year 1990, one in every 1000 children attaining the age of 20 would be a survivor of ALL. Peckham et al. (1988) were able to report that survivors of childhood cancer were more numerous among school-aged children in the USA than those who were severely and profoundly retarded, hard of hearing, deaf, or visually handicapped. As noted above, the five-year survival rate of ALL in the 1990s has risen to 72.8% (Boring et al., 1991).

Subsequently, with such advances in treatment, ALL is no longer viewed as an almost invariably fatal disease, but as a life-threatening illness, with long-term disease-free survival frequently achieved, and cure as a realistic goal (Meadows et al., 1980; McCalla, 1985; Muchi et al., 1987). Undoubtedly, the development of effective treatments for ALL has been one of the resounding success stories in the area of oncology.

Treatment of leukaemia

Treatment of leukaemia is aimed at inducing, consolidating and maintaining remission of leukaemic cells, and involves the use of multiple cytotoxic drugs in complex protocols, with or without the administration of cranial irradiation. There is a dual approach to treatment: as ALL is fundamentally a disease of the blood, the primary treatment goal is to use drugs to destroy the blood-borne cancerous cells. The second treatment goal is to prevent the spread of these cells throughout the nervous system (Cousens et al., 1990). Regimens for the prevention of central nervous system (CNS) leukaemia vary, and usually consist of intrathecal chemotherapy, CNS irradiation and high-dose intravenous chemotherapy, or combinations of these approaches (Bleyer and Poplack, 1985; McWhirter and Masel, 1987).

Chemotherapy is the treatment of cancerous conditions by chemical agents or drugs. Drug administration for the treatment of childhood cancer was first reported in the late 1940s by Farber and colleagues (Farber et al., 1948). Although in the early years of chemotherapy, cytotoxic drugs were usually administered as single agents, in more recent times, to heighten the effect of the drugs, chemotherapy has generally involved the administration of a combination of drugs (McWhirter and Masel, 1987).

Radiotherapy is the treatment of disease using ionizing radiation. The use of radiation as a treatment modality was first attempted in the late nineteenth century, and followed closely on the discovery of X-rays by

Roentgen, radioactivity by Becquerel, and radium by the Curies (Kaplan, 1975). During the treatment process, tissues containing neoplastic cells are exposed to beams of radiation. Because cancer cells are particularly sensitive to radiation, their rapid multiplication is controlled, and ultimately, the abnormal cells are destroyed, while the surrounding normal tissue remains relatively intact. Much research, however, has been aimed at determining the maximum amount of radiation that can be delivered before damage to normal tissue is induced (Marks et al., 1981; Marks and Wong, 1985). Nevertheless, despite advances in research, damage to normal tissue as a result of irradiation is still frequently documented. As part of a course of radiotherapy, radiation can be administered to any body part containing either benign or malignant neoplastic cells. The amount of radiation used varies, depending on the nature of the neoplasm. The unit of measurement representing the absorbed dose of ionizing radiation is a 'rad' (radiation absorbed dose).

Induction therapy

According to Miller (1982), there are three aims of the induction of remission in acute lymphoblastic leukaemia. These are:

- To destroy as many leukaemic cells as rapidly as possible.
- To preserve normal haematopoietic cells.
- To restore haematopoiesis (production of red blood cells) as quickly as possible.

Remission has been reported to occur in 85% of children with acute lymphoblastic leukaemia when treated with two cytotoxic drugs (usually vincristine and prednisone) in combination (Poplack and Reaman, 1988). An even better remission rate of 95% has been reported when a third agent (e.g. L-asparaginase) is added to the treatment protocol (Miller, 1982). However, because treatment protocols containing four or more active agents are associated with a higher incidence of complications and toxicity during induction, they are used only in the treatment of cases with a poor prognosis (Hughes et al., 1975).

The use of chemotherapy is constantly changing and being revised. By the 1970s, chemotherapy was successful in maintaining haematological remission for extended periods in many children diagnosed with ALL. However, relapses and an eventual terminal phase occurred in the majority that were resistant to further chemotherapy (Said et al., 1989). Death in the course of ALL principally results not from the original disease of the blood, but from the infiltration of the CNS by blast cells.

Consolidation therapy

Children with ALL are at risk of developing CNS leukaemia (Littman et al., 1987). The blood–brain barrier, while protecting the CNS by monitoring the chemicals allowed to enter the CNS, does not offer adequate protection from the infiltration of leukaemic cells. Moreover, systemic chemotherapy has no effect on leukaemic cells present in the CNS, since the therapeutic agents cannot cross the blood–brain barrier to gain access to the invading leukaemic cells.

Consequently, the CNS acts as a sanctuary site for leukaemic cells, which are then able to proliferate and eventually metastasize to the bone marrow and other peripheral sites, thus 're-seeding' the bone marrow with leukaemic cells, and thereby causing a systemic relapse. Without prophylaxis to prevent overt leukaemic infiltration of the CNS, many children who initially survive ALL eventually develop CNS leukaemia, which is difficult to eradicate, causes considerable discomfort, and is associated with a risk of further neurological complications (Chessells, 1985a; Ochs et al., 1985).

The incidence of CNS leukaemia in children with ALL is considerably reduced by adequate presymptomatic prophylaxis (CNS prophylaxis), which involves administration of cranial irradiation in conjunction with intrathecal methotrexate (MTX) (Kim et al., 1972; Hustu and Aur, 1978; Sposto and Hammond, 1985). Intrathecal chemotherapy involves the injection of drugs through the theca of the spinal cord into the subarachnoid space and can consist of MTX, cytosine arabinoside, or hydrocortisone. In fact, the risk of developing CNS leukaemia can be reduced from as high as 50–60% in children receiving minimal or no prophylactic CNS treatment (Green et al., 1980; Moe, 1984; Littman et al., 1987; Ludwig et al., 1987) down to 3–10% by administering prophylactic cranial irradiation and intrathecal MTX during the early phases of consolidation therapy, when no signs of CNS leukaemia are actually present (Pinkel, 1979; Ch'ien et al., 1981; Moe, 1984; Chessells, 1985b; Kaleita and Al-Mateen, 1985; Littman et al., 1987). CNS radiotherapy for ALL is administered to a total dose of 1800 to 2400 rads, usually in daily fractions of 180 to 200 rads until the total dose specification has been reached.

CNS prophylaxis is vital because the infiltration of leukaemic cells into the CNS is not readily detectable by current diagnostic procedures (Madan-Swain and Brown, 1991). Although the need for CNS prophylaxis is unquestionable, evidence has accumulated which suggests that this therapy may be associated with adverse long-term sequelae (Moss et al., 1981). The increase in the number of survivors of ALL has led to the recognition of some of these important late sequelae of the disease and its treatment (McWhirter et al., 1986). With improvement in survival, especially for children with the most favourable outlook, there has been a shift in emphasis, with almost as much concern shown for the late effects of treatment as for the improvement of present therapy itself (Esseltine et al., 1981; Meadows et al., 1981; Rodgers et al., 1991), such that, according to Rodgers et al. (1991), the management philosophy has progressed from 'cure at almost any cost' to 'cure at least cost'. Among the late consequences of CNS prophylaxis are structural and functional changes in the brain and a range of adverse late cognitive sequelae, which are discussed further in Chapter 2.

Maintenance therapy

Maintenance chemotherapy is also an essential part of the treatment of children with ALL. Without some form of maintenance therapy, remission in most patients lasts only one to two months (Frei, 1965). As in the case of remission induction, most maintenance therapy programmes employ a multiple drug regimen. The choice of drugs varies according to different risk groups. For example, a multiple agent regimen may involve reinforcement chemotherapy with periodic (i.e. monthly or quarterly) chemotherapy pulses. The two most frequently administered drugs in reinforcement therapy are MTX (administered weekly or twice weekly) and 6-mercaptopurine (administered daily). In addition, remission appears to be prolonged by intermittent pulses of vincristine and prednisone, with or without L-asparaginase. It must be noted, however, that pulsed chemotherapy may not be required for all patients (Fernbach et al., 1975; Simone, 1976; Rivera and Mauer, 1987). As in remission induction, it has been found that, although multiple drug regimens are superior to single drug treatments for the purpose of maintenance therapy, adding too many chemotherapeutic agents to the protocol merely serves to increase the toxicity and morbidity associated with the treatment, without having any significant effect on remission duration or survival in most patients (Haghbin, 1976; Aur et al., 1978b), except perhaps for those with a very poor prognosis.

Paediatric brain tumours

Types of posterior fossa tumour

Brain tumours are a recognized cause of acquired speech and language disorders in childhood (Brown, 1985; Rekate et al., 1985; Volcan et al., 1986; Ammirati et al., 1989; Hudson et al., 1989; Murdoch and Hudson-Tennent, 1994a, b). As indicated earlier, however, the nature and distribution of brain tumours differs in children compared to adults, with tumours in the posterior cranial fossa accounting for the majority of all paediatric intracranial neoplasms. The most common posterior fossa tumours are medulloblastomas, astrocytomas and ependymomas. Based on a sample of 151 children with posterior fossa tumour, Menkes and Till (1995) reported that 34.4% had medulloblastomas, 21.9% had astrocytomas and 10.6% ependymomas. Brainstem neoplasms were present in 26.5% of the 151 cases. Similar figures for the occurrence of various posterior fossa tumours were reported by Matson (1956). The major characteristics of medulloblastomas, astrocytomas and ependymomas are summarized in Table 1.1.

Table 1.1 Characteristics of medulloblastomas, astrocytomas and ependymomas

Feature	Medulloblastoma	Astrocytoma	Ependymoma
Malignancy*	Highly malignant	Grades I–IV	Grades I–IV
Age at onset	4 m – 16 y	0–16 y	0–7 y
Male/female ratio	1.3:1	1:1	Reports vary
Incidence (%)**	34.4	21.9	10.6
Origin	Cerebellar vermis	Cerebellar hemisphere	Fourth ventricle
Symptom duration***	1–80 m	2 y 4 m	Unreported
Medical prognosis	Variable	Favourable	Variable
Tumour recurrence	10–100% of cases reported	Rare	Common
Symptoms	Headache, nausea, vomiting, gait disturbance, apathy, irritability, neck stiffness/pain, dizziness, papilloedema, squint, nystagmus, change in muscle tone, tendon reflex changes, dorsiflexor plantar response, head tilting, visual impairment, limb paresis, facial weakness		

*Based on the Kernohan classification with Grade I being benign and Grade IV highly malignant.
**Proportion of paediatric posterior fossa tumour cases diagnosed by Menkes and Till (1995).
***Average symptom duration reported in 43 cases by Davis and Joglekar (1981).
y = years; m = months.

Medulloblastomas

Medulloblastomas are highly malignant brain tumours derived from primitive neurones, the neuroblasts. In particular, the majority of these tumours are thought to arise from embryonal cell nests in the posterior medullary velum of the cerebellum. Although these tumours originate from the cerebellum, they subsequently invade the subarachnoid spaces, fourth ventricle and spinal canal. As the tumour grows it tends to extend backwards and may occlude the foramen magnum and infiltrate the meninges. Most medulloblastomas are situated in the midline of the cerebellum (i.e. the vermis). Characteristically, on CT scans, medulloblastomas appear as relatively well-defined, non-calcified, non-cystic, slightly dense inferior vermian masses. Children have been diagnosed with medulloblastomas between four months and 16 years of age with there being a slightly higher (1.3:1) incidence in male children. The primary concern for patients with medulloblastomas is the risk of tumour recurrence in the posterior cranial fossa and/or the development of supratentorial, spinal cord or systemic metastases. Where they occur, recurrences usually arise in the first two to three years following treatment with an average survival time for patients with recurrence of only 19 months. The prognosis for patients with recurrent medulloblastoma is, therefore, poor. Currently, the overall five-year disease-free survival rate for medulloblastoma is approximately 50% for patients treated with surgery and craniospinal irradiation (Menkes and Till, 1995).

Factors which appear to influence the prognosis of children with medulloblastoma include:

- The extent of surgical resection of the tumour, with total removal resulting in a more favourable outlook than subtotal or partial resection, or biopsy (Raimondi and Tomita, 1979; Norris et al., 1981; Park et al., 1983; Rivera-Luna et al., 1987; Russell and Rubinstein, 1989).
- The amount of radiation administered [according to Russell and Rubinstein (1989), a dose of at least 5000 rads is required if treatment is to be effective].
- The inclusion of chemotherapy in the treatment protocol.

Recent controlled studies designed to evaluate the addition of chemotherapy to the medulloblastoma treatment programme have reported favourable progression-free survival rates when compared with treatment utilizing radiotherapy alone (Fossati-Bellani et al., 1984; Rivera-Luna et al., 1987; Packer et al., 1989). Optimistic results have, however, been qualified by the recognized need for long-term follow-up of the subjects studied to date. In addition, after studying a large cohort of 179 children (88 received radiochemotherapy, whereas 91 underwent radiotherapy only), Evans et al. (1990) concluded that the addition of chemotherapy to the medulloblastoma treatment protocol only benefited those with more advanced stages of disease. Finally, the occurrence of extraneural metastases subsequent to medulloblastomas implies a poor prognosis. Metastatic deposits are most frequently diagnosed in the lymph nodes and the bones (Campbell et al., 1984; Russell and Rubinstein, 1989).

Although medulloblastomas have a less favourable prognosis than astrocytomas, advances in management techniques are improving the long-term outlook of medulloblastoma patients. Tumour recurrence and metastatic spread can occur, however, despite surgery, radiotherapy and chemotherapy, and generally indicate a poor prognosis for long-term survival.

Astrocytomas

As the name implies, astrocytomas are derived from the astrocytic neuroglial cells. Although they can occur above or below the tentorium cerebelli, infratentorial astrocytomas are more common in children. These tumours, when located in the posterior cranial fossa, can arise from either the vermis or lateral lobes of the cerebellum and tend to be well-circumscribed and often cystic, containing one or more sacs of clear yellow or brown fluid. These tumours are amenable to complete surgical excision as brainstem invasion is rare (Delong and Adams, 1975). Malignant transformation (anaplasia) of cystic cerebellar astrocytomas is uncommon.

Eighty-two percent of the 75 cases of cerebellar astrocytoma reviewed by Gol (1963) were of the cystic type, whereas the remaining 18% were solid astrocytomas. Gol (1963) described three forms of cystic astrocytoma:

- A neoplastic cyst where the neoplasm lined all the walls of the cyst.
- A cyst where the walls consisted of non-malignant glial tissue with the tumour concentrated in a nodule of vascular tumour tissue protruding from the wall of the cyst.
- A tumour which is polycystic in nature.

Klein and McCullough (1985) also detailed three forms of astrocytoma:

- A tumour with a large cyst and a mural tumour nodule (most favourable for total surgical removal).
- A solid tumour containing small visible cysts.
- A uniformly solid tumour.

Solid tumours are more frequently positioned in the midline, and are therefore associated with an increased risk of brainstem involvement. Solid tumours may display diffusely infiltrative edges, and are particularly prone to anaplastic changes and recurrence in adult patients. Fortunately, 68–86% of childhood cerebellar astrocytomas are cystic in nature (Gol and McKissock, 1959; Gol 1963; Lee et al., 1989).

As well as being described as cystic or solid, astrocytomas are also referred to as either juvenile or diffuse. Juvenile astrocytomas, as their name suggests, tend to appear during the first decade of life, whereas diffuse astrocytomas usually arise in adolescence. Juvenile astrocytomas

are compact, clearly demarcated tumours; diffuse astrocytomas infiltrate the surrounding brain tissue and are more prone to anaplastic
change than the juvenile type. Juvenile and diffuse forms of astrocytoma are not directly correlated to the cystic and solid types discussed
earlier (Gjerris and Klinken, 1978). Approximately 75% of childhood
cerebellar astrocytomas are of the juvenile type, the remaining 25%
being diagnosed as diffuse (Gjerris and Klinken, 1978; Davis and
Joglekar, 1981).

Astrocytomas are usually assigned a grade from I to IV according to
their level of malignancy, with grade I being benign and grade IV highly
malignant. Most cerebellar astrocytomas are low grade and, therefore,
associated with a favourable prognosis post-surgical removal (Gol and
McKissock, 1959; Naidich and Zimmerman, 1984; Kadota et al., 1989).
However, grade III and IV astrocytomas do occur and are referred to as
'glioblastomas'. Glioblastomas are rare in the cerebellum and spinal
cord (Koh et al., 1985). Despite the existence of some more malignant
forms of astrocytoma, tumour recurrence although reported is rare.
Complete surgical excision of astrocytomas, however, may be limited by
brainstem involvement and malignancy (Klein and McCullough, 1985).
According to Klein and McCullough (1985), the degree of brainstem
involvement and the level of malignancy place greater restrictions on the
surgical removal of cerebellar tumours than the size of the tumour, in
that relatively extensive resection of cerebellar tumours can be
performed with minimal functional loss.

In general, therefore, recovery from astrocytomas is favourable,
particularly when the tumour does not involve the brainstem, has a low
grade of malignancy, and complete surgical resection is possible.

Geissinger and Bucy (1971) reported the average age at diagnosis of
cerebellar astrocytoma to be eight years and nine months. However,
children presenting with this type of tumour at clinics for treatment of
associated dysarthria could be expected to vary in age from infancy
through to adolescence. Males and females appear to be affected equally.

Ependymomas

Ependymomas are slow-growing, predominantly benign neoplasms
derived from the ependymal cells lining the ventricles of the brain.
Although they can arise from any part of the ventricular system, the
roof and the floor of the fourth ventricle are the most common origins
for ependymomas in children. From there, the tumour grows to
occlude the cavity of the fourth ventricle, protrudes into the cisterna
magna or may extend through the foramen magnum to overlap the
cervical segments of the spinal cord. Due to their origins in the roof or
floor of the fourth ventricle, however, complete surgical resection is
not possible so that recurrence of the tumours in the primary site is

common. Development of metastases in other sites, however, is unusual. Tumour recurrence rates as high as 90% have been reported (Menkes and Till, 1995). If tumour recurrence does occur, it is usually identified within four years of the initial diagnosis (Salazar et al., 1983).

Five-year survival rates of 39% and 40.7% were reported by Naidich and Zimmerman (1984) and Nazar et al. (1990), respectively. However, others have determined far more favourable survival rates. For example, Salazar et al. (1983) calculated 10-year survival rates of 75% for grades I and II ependymomas and 67% for grades III and IV tumours in a group of 51 children and adults treated with surgery and radiotherapy for either infratentorial (31 patients) or supratentorial (20 patients) ependymomas. Similarly, Ross and Rubinstein (1989) described 15 patients with malignant ependymomas (10 were situated in the posterior fossa) and found 10 patients (67%) to be alive from 15 months to 14 years after surgery. Bloom et al. (1990) reported five-, 10- and 15-year survival rates of 51%, 40% and 31%, respectively, in a group of 51 children. Bloom and co-workers also observed an increasing five-year survival rate with increasing age at diagnosis. Overall, the prognosis for a child with an ependymoma is poor in terms of ultimate cure.

Brainstem tumours

In addition to the more common posterior fossa tumours outlined above, children can also experience a variety of brainstem tumours. The initial presentation of brainstem tumours in children varies from case to case. All, however, show a uniformly fatal progression. The tumours themselves may vary from benign astrocytomas through to highly malignant glioblastomas. The majority are in general malignant and arise from the pons. Manifestations of brainstem tumours in children appear at two to twelve years of age with a peak incidence at six years. Neurological signs may include cranial nerve palsies (including associated speech disturbances if cranial nerves supplying the speech production mechanism are involved), pyramidal tract signs and cerebellar signs. Vomiting and disturbances of gait are the most common presenting complaints. Cranial nerves most commonly affected are nerves VII and VI, with the facial weakness being of the lower motor neurone type and associated with a degree of flaccid dysarthria. Other cranial nerves may also be affected with increasing numbers involved over time. Progression of symptoms is relentless with patients becoming unable to speak (anarthric) or swallow, and the extremities becoming paralysed. Eventually, damage to the reticular formation, cardiac and respiratory centres leads to cardiac and respiratory problems, coma and death. Average survival time post-initial hospital admission is 15 months (Panitch and Berg, 1970).

Clinical symptoms of posterior fossa tumours

The presenting signs and symptoms of any posterior fossa tumour type are largely due to increased intracranial pressure which results from the mass effect of the tumour itself, associated oedema and obstruction to the flow of cerebrospinal fluid. Destruction or compression of brain tissue may also underlie many of the signs and symptoms observed (Tew et al., 1984). Symptoms associated with the presence of a brain tumour may be non-specific or localizing. Non-specific symptoms (e.g. headache, nausea) could be caused by many other childhood illnesses and do not necessarily suggest neurological damage, whereas localizing symptoms (e.g. ataxia, nystagmus) imply nervous system involvement.

Symptoms associated with posterior fossa tumours include bifrontal headache, nausea and vomiting, gait disturbance, depressed cerebral function (manifested as apathy and irritability), neck stiffness or neck pain, dizziness, papilloedema (oedema of the optic discs due to impairment of the venous drainage from the optic nerve and retina subsequent to increased intracranial pressure), squint and nystagmus, alteration of muscle tone, tendon reflex changes, dorsiflexor plantar response, tilting the head away from the side of the tumour, visual impairment, and paresis of limbs (Matson, 1956; Gol, 1963; Delong and Adams, 1975; Tew et al., 1984; Kadota et al., 1989). Facial weakness and deafness are rare but have been reported (Delong and Adams, 1975). Although seizures may be the presenting symptom in childhood supratentorial neoplasms (Hirsch et al., 1989), seizures have not been reported in association with tumours of the posterior fossa.

In that they share a cerebellar site, the clinical symptoms of medulloblastomas and astrocytomas are essentially the same. However, the duration between the onset of symptoms and initiation of treatment tends to be much shorter in the case of medulloblastomas (Delong and Adams, 1975), possibly due to the rapid growth of these tumours and the midline position of medulloblastomas. Both of these features result in the early obstruction of the fourth ventricle and interruption of the cerebrospinal fluid flow. The time between onset of symptoms and initiation of treatment in the case of medulloblastomas has been reported to average 5.2 months (range 1–80 months) whilst the same period for astrocytoma patients is two years four months (Davis and Joglekar, 1981). In general, the symptoms associated with ependymomas cannot be distinguished from medulloblastomas and astrocytomas (Delong and Adams, 1975; Naidich and Zimmerman, 1984). However, as ependymomas block the flow of cerebrospinal fluid prior to invading the cerebellum the initial symptoms are those associated with increased intracranial pressure rather than cerebellar deficits.

Treatment of posterior fossa tumours

Treatment of posterior fossa tumours involves surgical removal of the tumour, supplemented in some cases by craniospinal irradiation and, in the case of highly malignant tumours, by chemotherapy. Whether craniospinal irradiation and chemotherapy are required is determined by the degree of surgical excision (i.e. whether the tumour has been totally or only partially removed) and the level of malignancy of the tumour.

Access to the posterior cranial fossa is gained by way of a craniotomy through the occipital region of the cranium. Macroscopically, tumour removal is judged as total, subtotal (at least 80% of the tumour is excised), or partial. If the tumour is inaccessible only a biopsy is taken to allow determination of the tumour type. The extent of tumour excision depends on the neurological deficits that are likely to result from aggressive surgical resection.

The tumour tissue removed at surgery is analysed and a histological diagnosis made. Subsequent treatment depends largely on the pathologist's report and the extent of the tumour resection. Most children receive whole brain and/or spinal irradiation with an extra boost to the tumour site. Children with low grade astrocytomas are often spared craniospinal irradiation, a factor which may lead to a lower incidence of neuropsychological sequelae, including speech and language disorders, in the long term (see Chapters 3, 4 and 8). A typical course of radiotherapy may consist of a total irradiation dose of 5000–6000 rads, which is administered in daily fractions of 180 rads until the total dose is reached. A course of radiotherapy takes approximately six weeks to complete. Completing a course of radiotherapy is a gruelling experience for both the child and the family. The child often feels tired, irritable and nauseous, whereas the family is required to spend many hours each week accompanying the child to the radiotherapy clinic.

Children with highly malignant tumours may also receive chemotherapy. Although post-operative chemotherapy is not administered as routinely as radiotherapy, it has been suggested that when added to a regimen of surgical excision and CNS irradiation, or when implemented in cases of recurrent tumour, chemotherapy will prolong survival time (Horowitz et al., 1988; van Eys et al., 1988). Chemotherapy protocols can vary widely in drug selection, dosages and timing. Both chemotherapy and radiotherapy courses, and the complications which may be associated with such treatments, are discussed in detail in Chapter 2.

As discussed previously, many patients experience tumour recurrence despite aggressive tumour management at initial diagnosis. Depending on the site and growth characteristics of the recurrent tumour, these patients undergo further surgery, radiotherapy and/or chemotherapy. In some cases, the additional treatment is described as palliative rather than curative, with the ultimate aim being the alleviation of symptoms and an extension of the expected survival time.

The majority of children with posterior fossa tumours experience hydrocephalus due to ventricular and cerebrospinal fluid pathway obstruction. This symptom is alleviated by the surgical insertion of a shunting system. The most common shunt utilized is a ventriculoperitoneal shunt, which drains fluid from the lateral ventricles into the peritoneal cavity. The shunting procedure is usually performed prior to surgical excision of the tumour, however, in some cases shunting may not be required until after the tumour has been resected.

Introduction to speech and language disorders in paediatric cancer

In recent years, it has become increasingly recognized that the treatments applied to various forms of paediatric cancer may be associated with a number of adverse, long-term sequelae that may negatively influence the quality of life of survivors of these conditions. Many of these negative sequelae are related to structural and functional changes in the brain induced by the treatment and include, among others, motor and sensory changes, cognitive deficits and speech/language disorders. For instance, CNS irradiation and chemotherapy, as used in the treatment of leukaemia and following surgical removal of posterior fossa tumours in order to prevent tumour spread or recurrence, have been reported to cause aphasia in some adults and intellectual deficits in some children (Bamford et al., 1976; Broadbent et al., 1981; Danoff et al., 1982; Duffner et al., 1983; Burns and Boyle, 1984; Silverman et al., 1984).

Language disorders have been reported to occur in children treated for ALL (Buttsworth et al., 1993; Murdoch et al., 1994), whereas both speech and language disorders have been observed in children following treatment for posterior fossa tumours (Hudson et al., 1989; Hudson and Murdoch, 1992; Murdoch and Hudson-Tennent, 1994a, b). Given the potential of a communication disorder to impede the child's future academic achievements, vocational opportunities and social interactions, it is important that health professionals, and especially speech/language pathologists, be aware that children treated for cancer may exhibit a range of communication deficits so that the appropriate preventative and remedial programmes can be established. To this end the speech and language disorders reported to occur in children treated for the most common forms of paediatric cancer are described and discussed in detail in subsequent chapters of this book.

References

Ammirati M, Mirzai S, Samii M (1989) Transient mutism following removal of a cerebellar tumour: a case report and review of the literature. Child's Nervous System 5: 12–14.

Ansel S, Nabemezi JS (1974) Two year survey of hematologic malignancies in Uganda. Journal of the National Cancer Institute 52: 1397–1401.

Aur RJA, Simone JV, Verzosa MS, Hustu HO, Barker LF, Pinkel DP, Rivera G, Dahl GV, Wood A, Stagner S, Mason C (1978a) Childhood acute lymphocytic leukemia: Study VIII. Cancer 42: 2123–2134.

Aur R, Simone J, Hustu O, Rivera G, Dahl G, Bowman P, George S (1978b) Multiple combination therapy for childhood acute lymphocytic leukemia (ALL). Blood 52 (Suppl. 1): Abstract No. 490: 238.

Bamford FN, Morris-Jones P, Pearson D, Ribeiro GG, Shalet SM, Beardwell CG (1976) Residual disabilities in children treated for intracranial space-occupying lesions. Cancer 37: 1149–1151.

Bleyer WA, Poplack DG (1985) Prophylaxis and treatment of leukemia in the central nervous system and other sanctuaries. Seminars in Oncology 12: 131–148.

Bloom HJG, Glees J, Bell J (1990) The treatment and long-term prognosis of children with intracranial tumours: a study of 610 cases, 1950–1981. International Journal of Radiation, Oncology, Biology, Physics 18: 723–745.

Boring CC, Squires TS, Tong T (1991) Cancer statistics, 1991. CA — A Cancer Journal for Clinicians 41: 19–36.

Broadbent VA, Barnes ND, Wheeler TK (1981) Medulloblastoma in childhood: long-term results of treatment. Cancer 48: 26–30.

Brown JK (1985) Dysarthria in children: neurologic perspective. In Darby JK (ed.) Speech and Language Evaluation in Neurology: Childhood Disorders. Orlando, FL: Grune & Stratton: 133–184.

Burns MS, Boyle M (1984) Aphasia after successful radiation treatment: a report of two cases (Letter to the Editor). Journal of Speech and Hearing Disorders 49: 107–111.

Buttsworth DL, Murdoch BE, Ozanne AE (1993) Acute lymphoblastic leukaemia: language deficits in children post-treatment. Disability and Rehabilitation 15: 67–75.

Campbell AN, Chan HSL, Becker LE, Daneman A, Park TS, Hoffman HJ (1984) Extracranial metastases in childhood primary intracranial tumours: a report of 21 cases and review of the literature. Cancer 53: 974.

Chessells JM (1985a) Cranial irradiation in childhood lymphoblastic leukaemia: time for reappraisal? British Medical Journal 291: 686.

Chessells JM (1985b) Risks and benefits of intensive treatment of acute leukemia. Archives of Disease in Childhood 60: 193–195.

Ch'ien LT, Rhomes JA, Verzosa MS, Coburn TP, Goff JR, Hustu HO, Price RA, Seifert MJ, Simone JV (1981) Progression of methotrexate-induced leukoencephalopathy in children with leukaemia. Medical and Pediatric Oncology 9: 133–141.

Cousens P, Ungerer JA, Crawford JA, Stevens MM (1990. The nature and possible causes of cognitive deficit after childhood leukaemia. Brain Impairment: Advances in Applied Research: Proceedings of the Fifteenth Annual Conference of the Australian Society for the Study of Brain Impairment: 173–181.

Crosley CJ, Rorke LB, Evans A, Nigro M (1978) Central nervous system lesions in childhood leukemia. Neurology 28: 678–685.

Danoff BF, Chowchock FS, Marquette C, Mulgrew L, Kramer S (1982) Assessment of the long-term effects of primary radiation therapy for brain tumours in children. Cancer 49: 1580–1586.

Davies JNP (1985) Leukemia in children in tropical Africa. Lancet ii: 65–67.

Davis CH, Joglekar VM (1981) Cerebellar astrocytomas in children and young adults. Journal of Neurology, Neurosurgery and Psychiatry 44: 820–828.

Delong GR, Adams RD (1975) Clinical aspects of tumours of the posterior fossa in childhood. In Vinken PJ, Bruijn GW (eds) Handbook of Clinical Neurology, Vol. 18: Tumours of the Brain and Skull, Part III. Amsterdam: North Holland: 387–411.

De Nully Brown P, Hertz H, Olsen JH, Yssing M, Scheibel E, Jensen OM (1987) Incidence of childhood cancer in Denmark 1943–1984. International Journal of Epidemiology 18: 546–555.

Duffner PK, Cohen ME, Thomas PRM (1983) Late effects of treatment on the intelligence of children with posterior fossa tumours. Cancer 51: 233–237.

Edington GM, Hendriske M (1973) Incidence and frequency of lympho-reticular tumours in Ibadan and the western state of Nigeria. Journal of the National Cancer Institute 50: 1623–1631.

Esseltine DW, Freeman CR, Chevalier LM, Smith R, O'Gorman AM, Dube J, Whitehead VM, Nogrady MB (1981) Computed tomography brain scans in long term survivors of childhood acute lymphoblastic leukemia. Medical Pediatric Oncology 9: 429–438.

Evans AE, Jenkin RDT, Sposto R, Ortega JA, Wilson CB, Wara W, Ertel IJ, Kramer S, Chang CH, Leikin SL, Hammond GD (1990) The treatment of medulloblastoma: results of a prospective randomized trial of radiation therapy with and without CCNU, vincristine, and prednisone. Journal of Neurosurgery 72: 572–582.

Farber S, Diamond LK, Mercer PD, Sylvester RF, Wolff JA (1948) Temporary remissions in acute leukemia in children produced by folic acid antagonist, 4-aminopteroyl-glutamic acid (aminopterin). New England Journal of Medicine 238: 787–793.

Farwell JR, Dohrmann GJ, Flannery JT (1977). Central nervous system tumours in children. Cancer 40: 3123–3132.

Fernbach DJ, George SL, Sutow WW, Rogab AH, Lane DM, Haggard ME, Lonsdale D (1975) Long-term results of reinforcement therapy in children with acute leukemia. Cancer 36: 1552–1559.

Fossati-Bellani F, Gasparini M, Lombardi F, Zucali R, Luccarelli G, Migliavacca F, Moise S, Nicola G (1984) Medulloblastoma: results of a sequential combined treatment. Cancer 54: 1956–1961.

Frei E (1965) Progress in treatment for the leukemias and lymphomas. Cancer 18: 1580–1584.

Geissinger JD, Bucy PC (1971) Astrocytomas of the cerebellum in children. Archives of Neurology 24: 125–135.

Gjerris F (1978) Clinical aspects and long-term prognosis of infratentorial intracranial tumours in infancy and childhood. Acta Neurologica Scandinavica 57: 31–52.

Gjerris F, Klinken L (1978) Long-term prognosis in children with benign cerebellar astrocytoma. Journal of Neurosurgery 49: 179–184.

Gol A (1963). Cerebellar astrocytomas in children. American Journal of Diseases of Childhood 106: 21–24.

Gol A, McKissock W (1959) The cerebellar astrocytomas: a report on 98 verified cases. American Journal of Neurosurgery 16: 287–296.

Green DM, Freeman AI, Sather HN, Sallan SE, Nesbut ME Jr, Cassady JR, Sinks LF, Hammond D, Frei E (1980) Comparison of three methods of central-nervous-system prophylaxis in childhood acute lymphoblastic leukaemia. Lancet i: 1398–1402.

Haghbin M (1976) Chemotherapy of acute lymphoblastic leukemia in children. American Journal of Hematology 1: 201–209.

Hirsch JF, Rose CS, Pierre-Kahn A, Pfister A, Hoppe-Hirsch E (1989) Benign astrocytic and oligodendrocytic tumours of the cerebral hemispheres in children. Journal of Neurosurgery 70: 568–572.

Holland JF, Glidewell O (1972) Chemotherapy of acute lymphoblastic leukemia of childhood cancer. Cancer 30: 1480–1487.

Hooper R (1975) Intracranial tumours in childhood. Child's Brain 1: 136–140.

Horowitz ME, Mulhern RK, Kun LE, Kovnar E, Sanford RA, Simmons J, Hayes A, Jenkins JJ (1988) Brain tumours in the very young child. Cancer 61: 428–434.

Hudson LJ, Murdoch BE (1992) Chronic language deficits in children treated for posterior fossa tumours. Aphasiology 6: 135–150.

Hudson LJ, Murdoch BE, Ozanne AE (1989) Posterior fossa tumours in childhood: associated speech and language disorders post-surgery. Aphasiology 3: 1–18.

Hughes WT, Feldman S, Aur RJA, Verzosa MS, Hustu O, Simone JV (1975) Intensity of immunosuppressive therapy and the incidence of pneumocystis carinii pneumonitis. Cancer 36: 2004–2009.

Hustu HO, Aur RJA (1978) Extramedullary leukemia. Clinical Hematology 7: 313–337.

Jackel CA, Murdoch BE, Ozanne AE, Buttsworth DL (1990) Language abilities of children treated for acute lymphoblastic leukaemia: preliminary findings. Aphasiology 4: 45–53.

Jacquillat C, Weil M, Gemon MF, Izrael V, Schaison G, Auclerc G, Ablin AR, Flandrin G, Tanzer J, Bussel A, Weisgerber C, Dresch C, Najean Y, Goudemand M, Seligmann M, Boiron M, Bernard J (1973) Evaluation of 216 four-year survivors of acute leukemia. Cancer 32: 286–293.

Kadota RP, Allen JB, Hartman GA, Spruce WE (1989) Brain tumors in children. Journal of Pediatrics 114: 511–519.

Kaleita TA, Al-Mateen M (1985) Case 36-1984: subacute necrotizing leukoencephalopathy after treatment for acute lymphocytic leukemia. [Letter to the Editor]. New England Journal of Medicine 312: 317.

Kaplan HS (1975) Present status of radiation therapy of cancer: an overview. In Becker FF (ed.) Cancer: A Comprehensive Treatise, Vol 6: Radiotherapy, Surgery, Immunotherapy. New York: Plenum: 3–38.

Kim R, Nesbit ME, D'Angio GD, Levitt SH (1972) The role of central nervous system irradiation in children with acute lymphoblastic leukemia. Radiology 104: 635–641.

Klein DM, McCullough DC (1985) Surgical staging of cerebellar astrocytomas in childhood. Cancer 56: 1810–1811.

Koh SJ, Brown RE, Simmons JCH (1985) Glioblastoma in children. Pediatric Pathology 4: 67–79.

Koocher GP, O'Malley JE (1981) Implications for patient care. In Koocher GP, O'Malley JE (eds) The Damocles Syndrome: Psychological Consequences of Surviving Childhood Cancer. New York: McGraw-Hill: 164–178.

Lannering B, Marky I, Nordborg C (1990) Brain tumors in childhood and adolescence in West Sweden 1970–1984. Cancer 66: 604–609.

Lee YY, Van Tassel P, Bruner JM, Moser RP, Share JC (1989) Juvenile pilocytic astrocytomas: CT and MR characteristics. American Journal of Neuroradiology 10: 363–370.

Littman P, Coccia P, Bleyer WA, Lukens J, Siegel S, Miller D, Sather H, Hammond D (1987) Central nervous system (CNS) prophylaxis in children with low risk acute lymphoblastic leukemia (ALL). International Journal of Radiation, Oncology, Biology, and Physics 13: 1443–1449.

Ludwig R, Calvo W, Kober B, Brandeis WE (1987) Effects of local irradiation and i.v. methotrexate on brain morphology in rabbits: early changes. Journal of Cancer Research and Clinical Oncology 113: 235–240.

Madan-Swain A, Brown RT (1991) Cognitive and psychological sequelae for children with acute lymphocytic leukemia and their families. Clinical Psychology Review 11: 267–294.

Marks JE, Baglan RJ, Prassad SC, Blank WF (1981) Cerebral radionecrosis: incidence and risk in relation to dose, time, fractionation and volume. International Journal of Radiation, Oncology, Biology and Physics 7: 243–252.

Marks JE, Wong J (1985) The risk of cerebral radionecrosis in relation to dose, time and fractionation. Progress in Experimental Tumour Research 29: 210–218.

Matson DD (1956) Cerebellar astrocytoma in childhood. Pediatrics 18: 150–158.

McCalla JL (1985) A multidisciplinary approach to identification and remedial intervention for adverse late effects of cancer therapy. Symposium on Pediatric Oncology 20: 117–130.

McWhirter WR, Masel JP (1987) Paediatric Oncology: An Illustrated Introduction. Sydney: Williams & Wilkins.

McWhirter WR, Pearn JH, Smith H, O'Reagan P (1986) Cerebral astrocytoma as a complication of acute lymphoblastic leukaemia. The Medical Journal of Australia 145: 96–97.

McWhirter WR, Petroeschevsky AL (1990) Childhood cancer incidence in Queensland, 1979–88. International Journal of Cancer 45: 1002–1005.

Meadows AT, Kreimas NL, Belasco JB (1980) The medical cost of cure: sequelae in survivors of childhood cancer. In Sullivan MP, van Eys J (eds) Status of the Curability of Childhood Cancers. New York: Raven: 263–276.

Meadows AT, Massari DJ, Ferguson J, Gordon J, Littman P, Moss K (1981) Declines in IQ scores and cognitive dysfunctions in children with acute lymphocytic leukaemia treated with cranial irradiation. Lancet ii: 1015–1018.

Menkes JH, Till K (1995) Postnatal trauma and injuries by physical agents. In Menkes JH (ed.) Textbook of Child Neurology. Baltimore: Williams & Wilkins: 557–597.

Miller DR (1980a) Acute lymphoblastic leukemia in children. Pediatric Clinics of North America 27: 269–291.

Miller DR (1980b) Childhood acute leukemia. In Conn HF (ed.) Current Therapy (32nd edition). St Louis: Mosby: 292–299.

Miller DR (1982) Acute lymphoblastic leukemia. In Tebbi CK (ed.) Major Topics in Pediatric and Adolescent Oncology. Boston: Hall Medical: 2–43.

Moe P (1984) Recent advances in the management of acute lymphoblastic leukemia. European Pediatric Haematology and Oncology 1: 19–28.

Moss HA, Nannis ED, Poplack DG (1981) The effects of prophylactic treatment of the central nervous system on the intellectual functioning of children with acute lymphoblastic leukemia. American Journal of Medicine 71: 47–52.

Muchi H, Satoh T, Kayoko Y, Karube T, Miyao M (1987) Studies on the assessment of neurotoxicity in children with acute lymphoblastic leukemia. Cancer 59: 891–895.

Murdoch BE, Boon DL, Ozanne AE (1994) Variability of language outcomes in children treated for acute lymphoblastic leukaemia: an examination of 23 cases. Journal of Medical Speech–Language Pathology 2: 113–123.

Murdoch BE, Hudson-Tennent LJ (1994a) Differential language outcomes in children following treatment for posterior fossa tumours. Aphasiology 8: 507–534.

Murdoch BE, Hudson-Tennent LJ (1994b) Speech disorders in children treated for posterior fossa tumours. European Journal of Disorders of Communication 29: 379–397.

Naidich TP, Zimmerman RA (1984) Primary brain tumours in children. Seminars in Roentgenology 19: 100–114.

Nazar GB, Hoffman HJ, Becker LE, Jenkin D, Humphreys RP, Hendrick EB (1990) Infratentorial ependymomas in childhood: prognostic factors and treatment. Journal of Neurosurgery 72: 408–417.

Neglia JP, Robison LL (1988) Epidemiology of the childhood acute leukemias. Pediatric Clinics of North America 35: 675–692.

Norris DG, Bruce DA, Byrd RL, Schut L, Littman P, Bilaniuk LT, Zimmerman RA, Capp R (1981) Improved relapse-free survival in medulloblastoma using modern techniques. Neurosurgery 9: 661–663.

Ochs JJ, Rivera G, Rhomes JA, Hustu HO, Berg R, Simone JV (1985) Central nervous system morbidity following an initial isolated central nervous system relapse and its subsequent therapy in childhood acute lymphoblastic leukemia. Journal of Childhood Oncology 3: 622–626.

Packer RJ, Sutton LN, Atkins TE, Radcliffe J, Bunin GR, D'Angio G, Siegel KR, Schut L (1989) A prospective study of cognitive function in children receiving whole-brain radiotherapy and chemotherapy: 2-year results. Journal of Neurosurgery 70: 707–713.

Panitch HS, Berg BD (1970) Brain stem tumours of childhood and adolescence. American Journal of Disorders of Childhood 19: 465–472.

Park TS, Hoffman HJ, Hendrick EB, Humphreys RP, Becker LE (1983) Medulloblastoma: clinical presentation and management. Journal of Neurosurgery 58: 543–552.

Parkin DM, Stiller CA, Draper GJ, Bieber CA (1988) The international incidence of childhood cancer. International Journal of Cancer 42: 511–520.

Peckham VC, Meadows AT, Bartel N, and Marrero O (1988) Educational late effects in long-term survivors of childhood acute lymphocytic leukemia. Pediatrics 81: 127–133.

Pinkel D (1979) Treatment of acute lymphocytic leukemia. Cancer 43: 1128–1137.

Poplack DG, Reaman G (1988) Acute lymphoblastic leukemia in childhood. Pediatric Clinics of North America 35: 903–932.

Raimondi AJ, Tomita T (1979) Medulloblastoma in childhood: comparative results of partial and total resection. Child's Brain 5: 310–328.

Rekate HL, Grubb RL, Aram DM, Hahn JF, Ratcheson RA (1985) Muteness of cerebellar origin. Archives of Neurology 42: 697–698.

Rivera GK, Mauer AM (1987) Controversies in the management of childhood acute lymphoblastic leukemia: treatment intensification, CNS leukemia, and prognostic factors. Seminars in Hematology 24: 12–26.

Rivera-Luna R, Reuda-Franco F, Lanche-Guevara MT, Martinez-Buerra G (1987) Multidisciplinary treatment of medulloblastomas in childhood. Child's Nervous System 3: 228–231.

Rodgers J, Britton PG, Kernahan J, Craft AW (1991) Cognitive function after two doses of cranial irradiation for acute lymphoblastic leukaemia. Archives of Disease in Childhood 66: 1245–1246.

Ross GW, Rubinstein LJ (1989) Lack of histopathological correlation of malignant ependymomas with postoperative survival. Journal of Neurosurgery 70: 31–36.

Russell DS, Rubinstein LJ (1989) Pathology of Tumours of the Nervous System (5th edition). London: Edward Arnold.

Said JA, Waters BGH, Cousens P, Stevens MM (1989) Neuropsychological sequelae of central nervous system prophylaxis in survivors of childhood acute lymphoblastic leukemia. Journal of Consulting and Clinical Psychology 57: 251–256.

Salazar OM, Castro-Vita H, Van Houtte P, Rubin P, Aygun C (1983) Improved survival in cases of intracranial ependymoma after radiation therapy: late report and recommendations. Journal of Neurosurgery 59: 652–659.

Segall HD, Batnitzky S, Zee S, Ahmadi J, Bird CR, Cohen ME (1985) Computed tomography in the diagnosis of intracranial neoplasms in children. Cancer 56: 1748–1755.

Silverman CL, Palkes H, Talent B, Kovnar E, Clouse JW, Thomas PRM (1984) Late effects of radiotherapy on patients with cerebellar medulloblastoma. Cancer 54: 825–829.

Simone JV (1976) Factors that influence haematological remission duration in acute lymphocytic leukaemia. British Journal of Haematology 32: 465–472.

Southam CM, Craver FL, Dargeon HW, Burchenal JH (1951) A study of the natural history of acute leukemia with special reference to the duration of the disease and the occurrence of remissions. Cancer 4: 39–59.

Sposto R, Hammond GD (1985) Survival in childhood cancer. Journal of Clinical Oncology 4: 195–204.

Tew JM, Feibel JH, Sawaya R (1984) Brain tumours: clinical aspects. Seminars in Roentgenology 19: 115–128.

Till MM, Hardisty RM, Pike MC (1973) Long survivals in acute leukaemia. Lancet i: 534–538.

Tivey H (1952) Prognosis for survival in the leukemias of childhood. Pediatrics 10: 48–59.

van Eys J, Baram TZ, Cangir A, Bruner JM, Martinez-Prieto J (1988) Salvage chemotherapy for recurrent primary brain tumours in children. Journal of Pediatrics 113: 601–606.

Volcan I, Cole GP, Johnston K (1986) A case of muteness of cerebellar origin. Archives of Neurology 43: 313–314.

Young JL, Miller RW (1975) Incidence of malignant tumors in US children. Journal of Pediatrics 86: 254–257.

Chapter 2
Effects of treatment for paediatric cancer on brain structure and function

BRUCE E MURDOCH, LISA J HUDSON AND
DEBORAH L BOON

Introduction

Significant improvements in the survival rates of children with various neoplastic conditions as a consequence of the development of more effective treatment techniques, has undoubtedly been one of the outstanding accomplishments of modern oncology. As described in Chapter 1, the treatment of childhood cancers usually involves the use of techniques such as radiotherapy and chemotherapy which, in the case of children with intracranial tumours, are administered in addition to surgical excision of the tumour. Unfortunately, over the past two decades, it has become increasingly recognized that, despite being essential for survival, both radiotherapy and chemotherapy may cause structural and functional changes in the central nervous system (CNS) leading to a number of long-term negative sequelae, which may include neuropsychological problems, sensory and motor deficits, and speech/language disorders (Bamford et al., 1976; Danoff et al., 1982; Silverman et al., 1984; Hudson and Murdoch, 1992a, b; Buttsworth et al., 1993; Murdoch and Hudson-Tennent, 1994 a,b). Given, therefore, that radiotherapy and chemotherapy are likely to be important factors contributing to the occurrence of communication impairments in children treated for cancer, the possible adverse effects of these two treatments are discussed in detail below.

Adverse effects of radiotherapy

The effects of irradiation on brain structure and function can be divided into acute reactions, early-delayed reactions and late-delayed reactions. Acute reactions comprise symptoms that arise during the course of radiotherapy. Early-delayed reactions appear from a few weeks to a few months after irradiation and tend to be only transient features. Late-delayed reactions, on the other hand, appear from several months to years after the completion of radiotherapy and tend to be progressive and more permanent in nature. Consequently, it is these latter reactions, to radiotherapy that are most likely to be associated with the occurrence of long-term speech/language disorders and will therefore, be the primary focus of attention in the present chapter. Included among the late-delayed reactions to radiotherapy is damage to both the grey and white matter of the brain, generalized cerebral and cerebellar atrophy, and damage to the vascular supply to the brain.

Grey matter damage following radiotherapy

Basal ganglia calcification (i.e. deposition of calcium in the tissue) has frequently been cited as a consequence of childhood cranial irradiation. Lee and Suh (1977) described two children who were irradiated at two years of age. Both children evidenced extensive bilateral calcifications in the basal ganglia at intervals of 10 and 14 years after radiotherapy. One child also had calcification of the thalamus, whereas the other had calcification of the cerebral cortex. Similarly, Pearson et al. (1983) identified basal ganglia calcification in three children who were also treated with radiotherapy when less than five years of age. In addition, calcification in the frontal and parietal lobes was also observed. Two older children studied by Pearson et al. (1983), aged nine and 11 years when irradiated, demonstrated slight dilation of the lateral ventricles, but no areas of calcification. Fourteen of the 49 children examined by Davis et al. (1986) had evidence of grey matter calcification. Lesions were most frequently noted at the junctions of grey and white matter, and in the basal ganglia, caudate nucleus and cerebellum.

Pontine calcifications have also been reported following cranial irradiation. The computerized tomographic (CT) scans of two children studied by Price et al. (1988) showed the presence of pontine calcifications nine months and 23 months post-irradiation. Basal ganglia calcifications and cortical atrophy were also evident. One patient (patient 2) had a repeat CT scan nine months after the initial scan which showed additional areas of calcification to be present, thereby suggesting that calcification occurring subsequent to irradiation may be progressive in nature.

White matter damage following radiotherapy

The two major forms of damage to the white matter reported to occur subsequent to radiotherapy include necrosis (i.e. changes in the neural tissue indicative of cell death) and calcification. Both specific and diffuse white matter damage has been reported to occur subsequent to radiotherapy and both adults and children have been identified as being affected (Marks et al., 1981; Lichtor et al., 1984).

Marks et al. (1981) described pathologically proven radionecrosis in seven adults. Reported sites of damage included the white matter of the right hemisphere, the white matter adjacent to the original tumour site, the white matter of both temporal lobes, the white matter of the occipital hemisphere opposite the original tumour and in the original tumour bed.

A 14-year-old male with internal capsule calcification following radiotherapy was described by Lichtor et al. (1984). Twelve years after the completion of irradiation, a large calcified mass in the right internal capsule and an area of increased density in the genu of the left internal capsule were identified by CT. Another 14-year-old boy examined by Yamashita et al. (1980) nine months following cranial irradiation demonstrated lesions within the deep white matter of both cerebral hemispheres. Grey matter damage was also diagnosed in this patient, with bilateral abnormalities being detected in the basal ganglia and cerebral peduncles. In addition to specific lesions, diffuse white matter damage following radiotherapy has also been reported by several investigators (Davis et al., 1986; Dooms et al., 1986).

Although white matter abnormalities have been identified in children who have experienced cranial irradiation, Tsuruda et al. (1987) failed to detect any lesions in 11 patients aged less than 20 years. These authors reviewed 95 patients who had received radiotherapy for CNS tumours. Magnetic resonance imaging (MRI) scans were viewed retrospectively and graded according to the changes involving white matter. Thirty-six of the 84 patients aged more than 20 years had symmetric white matter lesions remote from either the tumour or operative site. Relative sparing of the brainstem, cerebellum, internal capsules and basal ganglia was noted in these cases. Tsuruda et al. (1987) were unable to explain the absence of radiation-related damage in younger patients. The authors proposed that a follow-up interval used by them of less than two years for the younger patients may have antedated the appearance of any long-term changes. The older patients were assessed up to 71 months after the completion of irradiation.

White matter changes can be detected from five months to many years after the completion of radiotherapy. Doses of radiation that have been associated with alterations in white matter have reportedly ranged from 2340 to 6000 rads. No specific dose level has been suggested to increase the risk of white matter calcification or necrosis. Contrary to expectations, Marks et al. (1981) observed that white matter necrosis did not always occur in the region that received the highest radiation dose. Davis et al. (1986) attempted to link radiation dose and resultant damage, and found that children with white matter abnormalities had received between 2600 and 5000 rads, whereas those with calcifications had received between 3500 and 5500 rads, thereby suggesting that calcification is induced by slightly higher doses of radiation than other white matter abnormalities.

Brain atrophy following radiotherapy

Generalized atrophy of the cerebrum and cerebellum has been identified as a long-term sequelae of cranial irradiation. Davis et al. (1986), based on CT scans, diagnosed generalized atrophy of the brain in 25 of 49 children who had received cranial irradiation for primary CNS and/or skull-base tumours. The children studied by Davis et al. (1986) were aged from three months to 17 years when they received between 2600 and 5500 rads of CNS irradiation. Cerebral atrophy was also identified in four of the nine patients studied by Curnes et al. (1986), and in both children reported by Price et al. (1988). Cerebellar atrophy was also experienced by a 15-year-old described by Lichtor et al. (1984).

Cerebrovascular disease following radiotherapy

Using techniques such as arteriography, several researchers have documented changes in the cerebrovascular system subsequent to cranial irradiation. Painter et al. (1975) observed damage to the cerebrovascular system in four children after radiotherapy. The particular cerebrovascular damage reported included narrowing of the left internal carotid artery and the left ophthalmic artery, displacement of both the left anterior choroidal and posterior communicating arteries, stenosis of the right anterior and middle cerebral arteries, an elevated left middle cerebral artery, a stretched left anterior choroidal artery and severe atherosclerosis throughout the vertebrobasilar system.

On the basis of carotid angiography, Cantini et al. (1989) noted diffuse narrowing of the sylvian blood vessels and poor or no filling of the ascending frontal arteries in two children irradiated for supratentorial brain tumours. It is noteworthy also that both subjects also presented two and three years post-irradiation with aphasia and a transitory right hemiparesis.

Mechanisms of brain damage following radiotherapy

Currently, the mechanism by which radiotherapy induces changes in brain structure and function remains unknown. In an attempt to explain the actual effect of cranial irradiation on the brain, however, at least six different theories have been proposed. These theories are as follows:

1. Radiation damage represents primary injury to nervous tissue (Di Lorenzo et al., 1978).
2. Radiation adversely affects the rapid phase of myelination that occurs early in childhood (Davis et al., 1986). Davis and co-workers studied the CNS changes that occurred in 49 children given radiotherapy for brain tumours. The white matter abnormalities and the focal calcifications observed, in association with the fact that damage predomi-

nantly occurred in children less than three years of age, formed the basis for their hypothesis.

3. Radiation causes a transient abnormality in the biochemical mechanisms that maintain myelin (Nightingale et al., 1982). The failure of the nervous system to maintain myelin serves to explain the transient early-delayed reactions observed in recipients of cranial irradiation. This theory differs from that proposed by Davis et al. (1986), which deals with the more permanent interruption to myelination.

4. Radiation damage occurs secondary to vascular changes (De Reuck and vander Eecken, 1975; Kearsley, 1983; Curnes et al., 1986).

Curnes et al. (1986) proposed that demyelination occurs secondary to vascular changes. After using MRI to study nine patients with histories of radiotherapy, these investigators produced the following evidence to support their theory:

- A long interval following radiotherapy preceded the onset of symptoms.
- Fibrinoid changes occurred in arteriolar walls in the affected area.
- The most severe changes in the white matter occurred in deep locations adjacent to the ventricle where blood supply is most tenuous.
- A high correlation between the severity of vascular change and the severity of demyelination was determined.

De Reuck and vander Eecken (1975) also argued for a vascular aetiology in cases of radiation necrosis and demyelination. Thirteen autopsies were performed by these investigators on subjects with suspected radiation-related damage. Focal necrosis of the brainstem and of the cerebral hemispheres corresponded to the vascular territories of deep-perforating arteries. Diffuse necrosis and demyelination was predominant in the periventricular regions with sparing of the cortex and subcortical white matter. The periventricular lesions corresponded to the periventricular arterial border-zones. Arterial border-zones are highly susceptible to generalized disturbances of the cerebral blood flow. The sparing of the cerebral cortex and subcortical white matter was explained by the rich vascular supply of these structures due to leptomeningeal anastomoses.

Kearsley (1983) reported the late onset of cerebrovascular disease in two patients with histories of radiotherapy. In addition, he also presented an extensive literature review summarizing 35 cases of cerebrovascular disease following radiotherapy. Thirteen of the 35 patients described were children 12 years of age or younger. Damage to the cerebrovascular system included stenosis or occlusion of the internal carotid artery, the middle cerebral artery, the common carotid artery, the anterior cerebral artery or the vertebrobasilar artery. Changes were limited to the area irradiated and common presentations included headaches, aphasia and sudden hemiparesis or hemiplegia. Kearsley (1983) also noted the absence of reports of late cerebrovascular changes in children irradiated for acute lymphocytic leukaemia and suggested that the lower doses of irradiation (2000–4000 rads) administered to leukaemic patients may account for this observation.

Wright and Bresnan (1976), however, provided evidence to suggest that small amounts of radiation administered to young children can produce occlusion of large cerebral blood vessels. The child studied by Wright and Bresnan (1976) was only a few weeks old when she received 1000 rads over a two-month period to a hemangioma involving the left orbit. When six years of age she experienced two episodes of slow, slurred speech, confusion to questions, and a right hemiparesis without facial involvement. The symptoms cleared within one hour. Angiography showed a hypoplastic left carotid artery with occlusion of both the anterior and middle cerebral arteries. The authors attributed the transient symptoms to a transient low flow state in the affected areas of the brain.

The endothelial cell was considered to be the primary site of radiation damage by Martins et al. (1977). These investigators favoured the theory that damage to the cells lining the blood vessels leads to abnormal vascular permeability. This, in turn, allows the accumulation of plasma proteins in the vessel walls, which results in thickening and hyalinization of the vessels. Acute fibrinoid necrosis follows with possible rupturing of the blood vessels leading to oedema, necrosis and haemorrhaging, which present clinically as a cerebral mass effect.

5. Radiation damage represents an immune reaction. Irradiation promotes the synthesis of proteins with antigenic properties, which could then trigger a progressive allergic reaction in the host (Di Lorenzo et al., 1978). After reviewing the literature and studying two children with grey matter calcification, Lee and Suh (1977) claimed that an autoimmune reaction or hypersensitivity to radiation causes both vascular damage and demyelination. Grey matter calcification then develops as a result of the primary damage incurred.

6. White matter changes that follow irradiation represent the normal aging process but at an accelerated rate (Tsuruda et al., 1987). Tsuruda and co-workers reviewed 95 patients who had received radiotherapy for a wide variety of CNS tumours. The MRI scans of the irradiated patients were compared with those of 180 age-matched control subjects. The control subjects had no history of radiotherapy but had experienced benign or malignant intracranial lesions. Morphologically, the deep white matter changes in both groups had similar MRI scans. Both groups showed an increase in

changes with age, but these occurred at a greater rate in the irradiated group.

Neuropsychological, neurological and communication deficits following radiotherapy

Most studies that have examined the detrimental effects of cranial irradiation on cognitive, motor, sensory and communication abilities have examined these functions in children and adults treated for CNS tumours. Unfortunately, brain tumours are associated with a number of other complications (e.g. mass effect, blockage of cerebrospinal fluid circulation, interruption of blood supply etc.) that make it difficult to isolate radiotherapy as the sole cause of associated neuropsychological, behavioural and communication deficits. Despite this difficulty, however, cranial irradiation has frequently been implicated as a causal factor when cancer patients develop deficits in these areas subsequent to treatment.

Neuropsychological deficits following radiotherapy

Many authors have reported evidence of either below average IQ scores in irradiated populations (Danoff et al., 1982; Pearson et al., 1983; Copeland et al., 1985; Packer et al., 1989; Riva et al., 1989; Hoppe-Hirsch et al., 1990) or IQ scores that, although within normal limits, fell significantly below the score achieved by the control group/s used (Silverman et al., 1984; Riva et al., 1989). Scores that deteriorate as the time post-treatment elapses have also been reported (Silverman et al., 1984; Packer et al., 1989; Hoppe-Hirsch et al., 1990).

Learning disabilities resulting in impaired academic performance have been reported in children exposed to CNS irradiation. Varying educational abilities have been identified by several researchers ranging from mild deficits that require remedial assistance in the normal classroom setting to severe intellectual handicap requiring institutional or special school enrolment (Bamford et al., 1976; Broadbent et al., 1981; Deutsch, 1982; Copeland et al., 1985). Copeland et al. (1985) studied three groups of children who had received CNS chemotherapy. Only one of the groups (Group 2), however, had experienced CNS irradiation in addition to chemotherapy. The children in Group 2 performed significantly below those in Groups 1 and 3 on measures of arithmetic, block design, coding, written spelling, visual–motor integration, spatial memory and fine motor skills. Copeland et al. (1985) claimed that the children's language skills were within normal limits, however, this observation is doubtful given that it was based only on the results of three short semantic assessments. The language findings reported here in Chapters 3, 4 and 5 identify the need to determine the linguistic status of children treated with CNS irradiation by use of assessment procedures that are specifically designed to evaluate a wide range of linguistic skills.

The reported incidences of intellectual impairment subsequent to cranial irradiation range from 25 to 60%. Although the risk of children experiencing below average intelligence as a result of radiotherapy is widely recognized, it is also important that health professionals and parents are aware that, although a child treated for cancer with radiotherapy might have an intelligence quotient (IQ) that falls within the average range, their IQ post-treatment may actually be significantly below the pre-treatment level.

Other symptoms that have been noted in patients given radiotherapy for the treatment of brain tumours include:

- Confusion, poor concentration (Marks et al., 1981; Pearson et al., 1983).
- Poor or reduced memory capacity (Kun et al., 1983; Mulhern et al., 1986; Bendersky et al., 1988).
- Progressive dementia (Martins et al., 1977).
- Lethargy (Martins et al., 1977).
- Hyperactivity (Pearson et al., 1983; LeBaron et al., 1988).
- Headaches (Painter et al., 1975; Martins et al., 1977).
- Seizures (Painter et al., 1975; Marks et al., 1981; Hoppe-Hirsch et al., 1990).
- Behavioural problems (Mulhern et al., 1989).

Motor deficits following radiotherapy

Motor deficits have been reported to appear in some patients following radiotherapy. Ataxia, unsteady gait and limb inco-ordination are frequently recorded throughout the literature irrespective of the site of the original tumour (Bamford et al., 1976; Martins et al., 1977; Broadbent et al., 1981; Nightingale et al., 1982; Pearson et al., 1983; Silverman et al., 1984). In addition, Copeland et al. (1985) studied children with leukaemia or lymphoma and found that the 25 children in the irradiated leukaemia/lymphoma group demonstrated fine motor abilities that were significantly below those demonstrated by the non-irradiated leukaemia/lymphoma group and a group of children with solid tumours or Hodgkin's disease. This observation was made in the absence of the complicating factors often associated with tumours, giving further support to the reported link between ataxia and radiotherapy.

Spastic and flaccid hemiplegias of either the left or right sides of the body have also been reported in patients who have completed courses of radiotherapy (Painter et al., 1975; Bamford et al., 1976; Marks et al., 1981). Bamford et al. (1976) also noted the presence of cranial nerve palsies in 12 (40%) of the 30 patients reviewed at least five years after treatment for intracranial space-occupying lesions. Nerve palsies were the cause of squint in seven patients and facial weakness in four. Dysphagia due to a palatal weakness was experienced by one patient.

Thus, it appears that motor deficits can occur as a direct result of the radiotherapy administered in the treatment of cerebral tumours, leukaemia or lymphoma.

Sensory deficits following radiotherapy

Both visual and hearing impairments have been associated with radiotherapy given for the treatment of brain tumours. Painter et al. (1975) described an eight-year-old girl who developed bilateral optic atrophy and horizontal nystagmus four years four months after completing radiotherapy for a glioma of the optic chiasm.

Of the 30 long-term survivors of brain tumours reviewed by Bamford et al. (1976), 11 had correctable defects of acuity, whereas three experienced severe visual handicaps. Hearing impairments were detected in two of the 30 subjects (6.6%). One was described as partially deaf and the other as totally deaf. Severe hearing impairment was identified in four of the 73 (5%) medulloblastoma patients reviewed by Hoppe-Hirsch et al. (1990) five years' post-irradiation.

Communication disorders following radiotherapy

A number of studies reported in the literature have documented the occurrence of language disorders in children given radiotherapy as part of their treatment for paediatric cancer. A right hemiparesis and an aphasia were observed in a nine-year-old girl two years after partial resection of a cerebellar medulloblastoma and a course of radiotherapy by Painter et al. (1975). Chin and Maruyama (1984) attributed reading and writing difficulties, identified in six of their 10 subjects, to the radiotherapy given as part of the treatment for medulloblastoma. Similar observations were recorded by Packer et al. (1989) who reported a significant decline in the reading and spelling abilities of 14 children treated with radiotherapy for brain tumours that did not involve the cerebral cortex, subcortical white matter or deep grey masses.

More recently, Murdoch and colleagues, using a battery of specific linguistic tests, identified language problems in two different groups of children treated for cancer, including a group of children treated for posterior fossa tumours (Hudson et al., 1989; Hudson and Murdoch, 1992b; Murdoch and Hudson-Tennent, 1994a) and another group treated for acute lymphoblastic leukaemia (ALL) (Buttsworth et al., 1993; Murdoch et al., 1994). These studies represent the most extensive investigations of the language abilities of children treated for paediatric cancer reported to date and are the topics of major discussion in subsequent chapters of this book.

In addition to language disorders, communicative disorders in the form of dysarthria have also been reported to occur in children who have experienced irradiation to treat intracranial tumours. For example, two of the four subjects examined by Painter et al. (1975) exhibited facial paresis or dysarthria. All four subjects underwent cranial irradiation as children, and at the time of assessment showed evidence of cerebrovascular damage. A 29-year-old man described by Painter et al. (1975) demonstrated dysarthria, a flaccid right hemiparesis and difficulty with respiration 24 years after undergoing partial resection of a cerebellar medulloblastoma and receiving a total dose of 4800 rads to the posterior fossa and 3600 rads to the spine. The patient subsequently died and autopsy revealed severe atherosclerosis of the vertebrobasilar system, areas of encephalomalacia in the pons and medulla, and partial occlusion of the fourth ventricle by collagenous material. Painter et al. (1975) also reported the case of a young girl who received 2500 rads of radiation following removal of an optic chiasma tumour when she was eight months old. An additional 3500 rads was administered over four weeks when the child was aged 3;8. At eight years of age she had a right supranuclear facial paresis, a spastic right hemiparesis, bilateral optic atrophy and horizontal nystagmus.

Facial weakness was also identified in four of the 30 long-term survivors of childhood brain tumours examined by Bamford et al. (1976) with an additional subject demonstrating dysphagia associated with a palatal weakness. Murdoch and Hudson-Tennent (1994b) also reported the presence of a speech disorder in 11 of the 19 children treated for posterior fossa tumour included in their study. The findings of Murdoch and Hudson-Tennent (1994b) are the subject of detailed analysis in Chapter 8.

Adverse effects of chemotherapy

As outlined in the previous chapter, chemotherapy is used in a number of different ways in the treatment of childhood cancers. In conditions such as ALL, where there is no disease mass (tumour) present, chemotherapy may be the only form of treatment administered (see Chapter 1). In other conditions, chemotherapy may be given as an initial treatment in order to reduce the size of a large tumour. Chemotherapy is often administered subsequent to the surgical removal of an intracranial tumour from an infant. The growth of residual or recurrent tumours, and the risk of metastatic spread is controlled by use of chemotherapeutic drugs until the child is deemed old enough to tolerate a course of radiotherapy. The diagnosis of a high-grade tumour may prompt the instigation of combined radiochemotherapy post-surgery. Indeed, several authors have advocated such an approach in the treatment of medulloblastoma (Fossati-Bellani et al., 1984; Packer et al., 1986; Rivera-Luna et al., 1987). A more widespread practice is to reserve chemotherapy for cases evidencing recurrent disease following completion of the initial treatment programme involving surgery and radiotherapy. Furthermore, in those cases of childhood cancer that cannot be cured by chemotherapy, or indeed by any other form of treatment, chemotherapy is often used as a palliative therapy (i.e. a therapy aimed at alleviating without curing the disease).

Unfortunately, despite the many positive aspects of chemotherapy in the treatment of childhood cancer, in recent years a number of researchers have documented a possible link between chemotherapy and the occurrence of long-term negative side-effects, including alterations in brain structure and function, which in turn may be associated with declines in neurological and neuropsychological functioning. Although the difficulty inherent in distinguishing between the long-term side-effects of chemotherapy and those of radiotherapy has been acknowledged by the majority of researchers in the field, many authors have attempted to identify the detrimental effects of chemotherapy by studying children who are being treated for ALL. Whereas children with ALL may receive low doses of radiation (1800–2400 rads), it is claimed that chemotherapy, and in particular, intrathecal methotrexate (IT MTX), is the treatment variable under investigation.

There have been three principal classes of effect of CNS prophylaxis (for details of CNS prophylaxis see Chapter 1) identified in children with ALL (Cousens et al., 1990). The first involves physical damage to the brain, the second is damage to the endocrine system, and the third class of effect is impairment of cognitive functioning. Although the main thrust of this book is directed at speech/language impairment of survivors of paediatric cancer, it will be shown that it is not possible simply to isolate linguistic function and examine it as a separate entity, exhibiting no interaction with other factors. Interaction of factors is, of course, always operational in the social sciences, and never more so than in the case of a child treated for ALL who experiences the impact of complex and varied factors from all aspects of existence. These factors range from the effect of the treatment received to the family mechanism for coping with disease in one of its members. Hence, in attempting to focus ultimately on one aspect of an ALL survivor's functioning (i.e. linguistic functioning), it is essential that we are aware of the presence of other aspects contributing to that person as a whole (e.g. psychosocial elements, impact of CNS prophylaxis), in order to be able to take into consideration the possibility of such factors impinging on and interacting with one another. To that end then, all three classes of effect of CNS prophylaxis will be considered here.

Physical changes

Structural changes in the brain

Studies using CT scans and postmortem findings have identified a number of structural brain abnormalities in leukaemic patients who have received CNS prophylaxis. There are three types of structural changes in the brain that can occur subsequent to ALL treatment (Cousens et al., 1990):

- Leukoencephalopathy, which is destruction of the white matter (e.g. Price and Jamieson, 1975).
- Cortical atrophy, which is a wasting away of the grey matter of the cortex (Crosley et al., 1978).
- Microangiopathy, which is small blood vessel damage involving a calcification process and is often located in the basal ganglia (e.g. Price and Birdwell, 1978).

As Ochs and Mulhern (1988) pointed out, the actual clinical significance of CT scan changes remains unknown, and such changes should not be considered irreversible. Packer et al. (1986) drew attention to the more sensitive imaging obtainable using MRI, and suggested that such techniques are likely to increase the frequency and magnitude of structural CNS problems discovered. These authors anticipated that MRI will lead to more definite conclusions regarding the aetiology and pathogenesis of observed abnormalities.

Examples of leukoencephalopathy that have been documented from CT scans in children treated for ALL include focal areas of white matter hypodensity, ventricular dilation and cerebral calcifications (Day et al., 1978; Giralt et al., 1978; Peylan-Ramu et al., 1978; Kolmannskog et al., 1979; Obetz et al., 1979; Pizzo et al., 1979; Ochs et al., 1980, 1983, 1986; Allen et al., 1981; Esseltine et al., 1981; Habermalz et al., 1983; Pavlovsky et al., 1983; Brecher et al., 1985; Carli et al., 1985; Riccardi et al., 1985).

Another principal structural consequence of CNS prophylaxis is cortical atrophy (Di Chiro et al., 1988; Cousens et al., 1990). Findings of ventricular dilation and subarachnoid space dilation have been reported (e.g. Enzmann and Lane, 1978; Brouwers et al., 1985; Riccardi et al., 1985) and are thought to be indicative of cortical atrophy. Crosley et al. (1978) investigated 91 ALL subjects and found that cerebral atrophy was the most common lesion, occurring in 65% of the group. Furthermore, Crosley et al. (1978) reported that atrophy was most severe in subjects who were youngest at the time of diagnosis, or who had been treated with IT MTX alone or in combination with radiotherapy, or in whom duration of leukaemia was shortest.

Microangiopathies (calcification of cerebral blood vessels) have also been identified by a number of authors in patients treated with cranial radiation and IT MTX (e.g. Price and Birdwell, 1978; Ch'ien et al., 1981). Mineralizing microangiopathy, affecting the grey matter around the basal ganglia and adjacent subcortical areas, is a delayed neurotoxicity subsequent to CNS prophylaxis (Fletcher and Copeland, 1988). It has been proposed that radiotherapy is the agent causing microangiopathy, although it has also been suggested that MTX influences its development (McIntosh et al., 1977). There is also evidence that ALL children who are younger at the time of treatment may be more susceptible to lesions in the basal ganglia (Crosley et al., 1978; Price and Birdwell, 1978).

The findings of several postmortem investigations have also suggested that chemotherapy for the treatment of leukaemia might be responsible for inducing certain structural changes in the brain. Smith (1975) performed autopsies on 20 patients with ALL, acute myeloid leukaemia, hairy cell leukaemia, or non-Hodgkin's lymphoma. Ten had received IT MTX, whereas 10 patients were not given intrathecal therapy. Patients were between six months and 67 years of age at the time of diagnosis. Damage to the brain in patients given IT MTX included the destruction of oligodendroglial cells, white matter swelling, moderate to severe astrocytosis, petechial haemorrhages, oedema and coagulative necrosis. The damage was confined to the white matter of both the cerebrum and cerebellum. Although nine of the 10 patients given IT MTX also received up to 2400 rads of radiotherapy, Smith (1975) attributed the damage to the course of chemotherapy. She claimed that damage occurring in the brain following radiotherapy usually appeared many years after the conclusion of treatment. However, Smith (1975) failed to indicate the delay between the conclusion of chemotherapy and the detection of CNS damage in the 20 patients studied. In addition, it was claimed that the lesion types observed following the irradiation of intracranial tumours differed from those experienced by patients treated with chemotherapy for leukaemia. Smith (1975) described irradiation-related damage as being more severe and involving the cerebrovascular system. Although Smith (1975) recognized that the relatively low doses of irradiation used to treat patients with leukaemia might exacerbate the damage, it was concluded that MTX itself directly affects the oligodendrocyte.

Another case of intracranial damage following a course of IT MTX was reported by Skullerud and Halvorsen (1978). A two-year-old boy with leukaemia was administered IT MTX (6.5 mg per week for three weeks, followed by monthly injections of 6.5 mg). Radiotherapy was not given in this case. Twenty-four hours after completing the fifth IT MTX treatment, the child developed progressive flaccid paresis. Mental deterioration was observed and he died 18 days after the onset of the symptoms. Autopsy revealed areas of incomplete necrosis with astrocytosis on the base of the brain and along the insula, around the foramina of Luschka and over the superior and inferior colliculi. Similar lesions were also found over the surface of the cerebellum, particularly over the vermis. In contrast to the findings of Smith (1975), there were no lesions in the central white matter of the brain or spinal cord, or along the ependyma of the ventricles. It was concluded that MTX alone caused the lesions observed, because MTX was the only drug the patient received intrathecally, and, as tests showed no evidence of leukaemia within the CNS, the cancer could not have caused the damage. Skullerud and Halvorsen (1978) also noted that the most extensive tissue destruction occurred in areas that were in direct contact with the cerebrospinal fluid, and therefore with MTX.

Some studies record a high frequency of calcifications following CNS prophylaxis for ALL (McIntosh et al., 1977; Carli et al., 1985). Such findings emphasize the fact that the interaction between irradiation and subsequent IT MTX is, as yet, poorly understood (Carli et al., 1985; Ochs and Mulhern, 1988). Calcifications, which were originally ascribed to MTX, are yet to be reported in subjects who did not also receive irradiation (Ochs and Mulhern, 1988).

Despite the claims that MTX has negative effects on the structure and function of the nervous system, two studies involving relatively large patient groups failed to detect any long-term damage to the CNS. Ochs et al. (1980) examined 43 children with ALL. Ten patients were given IT MTX, whereas 33 received IT MTX in combination with intravenous MTX. All patients received weekly oral MTX. Patients were assessed using CT between 10 and 59 months (median = 29 months) after completion of treatment. It was concluded that none of the 43 patients had evidence of intracerebral calcification or areas of decreased attenuation (i.e. hypodense areas) on their CT scans. Although mild ventricular dilatation and visualization of the cortical sulci was detected in four patients, such features were also observed in control subjects.

Not many longitudinal investigations into structural changes to the brain following treatment for ALL have been performed, so the duration and course of such changes is generally unknown. Riccardi et al. (1985) proposed that, whereas ventricular dilatation may be mild and perhaps reversible, calcifications may increase in frequency and severity with time. Similarly, Ochs et al. (1983) suggested that hypodensity of the white matter may also be reversible.

Ochs and Mulhern (1988) surveyed a number of the existing CT studies in the literature and found a high frequency of cerebral calcifications, and pointed out that there is a wide range in the frequency of the structural changes seen in the various series of children in complete continuous remission. Ochs and Mulhern (1988) suggested that the wide range reflected not only the varied protocols used for CNS prophylaxis and systemic therapy but also the variable criteria used by different authors in classification of what constitutes a neurological 'change', as well as the variable follow-up times in each study. Beside the variety of constituents of CNS prophylaxis, another factor thought to contribute to the variability of the frequency and type of CT findings in ALL children was the age at the time of treatment. Some authors were of the opinion that a younger age at time of treatment has an adverse influence on CT findings (e.g. Carli et al., 1985; Riccardi et al., 1985), whereas other authors expressed a converse opinion, reporting more structural changes in older children (Habermalz et al., 1983).

Despite CT scans revealing lesions or neurological abnormalities following CNS prophylaxis, Cousens et al. (1988) pointed out that they often do not correlate with cognitive deficits (Paolucci and Rosito, 1983; Poplack, 1983; Harten et al., 1984). Only one group of researchers has published a positive correlation between structural and functional CNS changes. Brouwers et al. (1985) reported a positive relationship between ventricular dilatation and verbal fluency defects, and also between calcifications and memory deficits.

Besides causing physical changes to the structure of the brain, CNS prophylaxis can be linked with associated problems in the nervous system. These changes are discussed in the following section.

Neurological changes

Neurological problems are those resulting from disorders in the nervous system. CNS treatment of ALL is associated with a variety of neurological symptoms, with frequent reports of somnolence syndrome, which is characterized by sleepiness, anorexia, ataxia and other CNS dysfunctions (Freeman et al., 1973; Bleyer and Griffin, 1980). Somnolence syndrome occurs in 60% of leukaemic patients treated with radiotherapy, and is transient, with no clear-cut relation to long-term deficits (Fletcher and Copeland, 1988).

Delayed neurotoxicities are also possible following CNS prophylaxis. Leukoencephalopathy (whose physical manifestation in the brain has been discussed earlier) typically emerges several months after CNS prophylaxis, and is characterized by a slow onset of dementia, speech difficulties and other signs of deteriorating neurological status. It is thought that the incidence and severity of leukoencephalopathy is dependent on the amount and timing of radiotherapy and CNS chemotherapy (Fletcher and Copeland, 1988). Leukoencephalic lesions found in autopsy studies are generally white matter alterations in both hemispheres, thus indicating myelin degeneration.

Progressive dementia was observed by Pizzo et al. (1976) in a six-year-old girl undergoing a course of IT MTX without radiotherapy for relapse of meningeal leukaemia. The patient was disoriented to time and place, demonstrated a gait disturbance, and experienced a significant deterioration in reading and arithmetical abilities. IT MTX was discontinued and during the next six months the symptoms disappeared completely. The authors surmised that the lack of radiotherapy in this case eliminated the possibility that alteration of the blood–brain barrier enhanced the toxicity of IT MTX.

McIntosh et al. (1976) assessed 23 children who had received radiotherapy as part of their CNS prophylaxis of ALL, and found that although 11 subjects retained normal neurological function, the remaining children demonstrated neurological abnormalities. These 12 subjects developed mild, intermittent limping and a lack of co-ordination, which for six of the children progressed to include ataxia, seizures, hyperkinesis and learning disabilities.

Meadows and Evans (1976) also attributed the neurological symptoms observed in patients treated for leukaemia to MTX administered to the CNS. Four of the 23 children assessed by Meadows and Evans (1976) demonstrated severe impairments, including spastic quadriplegia or paraplegia and limited responsiveness. It is questionable that the symptoms were due solely to MTX, however, since three of the four severely impaired children also received up to 3400 rads of irradiation.

Five of the children assessed by Meadows and Evans (1976) demonstrated mild neurological dysfunction. Two had abnormal psychological test results and three required special education. Of the five patients showing minimal neurological deficits, three were given radiotherapy. However, it was claimed that in two cases the administration of radiation followed the signs of minimal cerebral dysfunction. Five of the 23 children examined by these workers had EEG abnormalities but were clinically asymptomatic. Nine patients had no signs of neurological abnormalities. These nine patients did not receive cranial irradiation, suggesting that MTX should not be cited as the sole cause of CNS damage in this study.

Meadows and Evans (1976) observed that the only clinical feature common to the 14 patients with some degree of neurological impairment was the administration of MTX in high doses (5–10 mg/kg per month) over prolonged periods (two to seven years). Although it was postulated that radiation may cause changes in the blood-brain barrier, allowing MTX to diffuse more easily into the white matter, the authors concluded that even MTX alone does have a direct effect on the nervous system, as not all of their patients had received radiotherapy. However, in order to isolate the elements that may contribute to any long-term deficits, it was recommended that patients receive detailed neurological and psychological examinations before, and at regular intervals after, CNS prophylaxis.

Endocrine changes

Another iatrogenic effect of CNS prophylaxis is damage to the endocrine system, with a deficit of growth hormone and retarded growth documented (Bamford et al., 1976; Kirk et al., 1987; Civin, 1989; Waber et al., 1990) and gonadal dysfunction a possibility that has, as yet, been only cursorily investigated (Ochs and Mulhern, 1988). It has been proposed that abnormalities of hypothalamic pituitary function are likely to be secondary to cranial irradiation, whereas gonadal dysfunction is probably secondary to chemotherapy (Ochs and Mulhern, 1988; Meadows et al., 1989). Anthropometric measurements commonly made in children for ALL include height, weight and head circumference. Microcephaly, short stature (growth retardation) and being overweight are frequent findings reported in the literature (e.g. Sainsbury et al., 1985; Kirk et al., 1987; Peckham et al., 1988; Waber et al., 1990). Adjectives frequently used to describe ALL survivors can include 'heavy', 'stocky', 'chubby', 'well-built' or 'obese' (Peckham et al., 1988).

Certain authors have found that growth is more impaired in girls than boys (Zurlo et al., 1988; Waber et al., 1990). Chessells (1983) stated that the possible factors resulting in impaired growth in children treated for ALL are cranial irradiation, spinal irradiation or long-term chemotherapy. However, despite possible abnormalities of growth hormone secretion, the majority of children with ALL have a normal growth pattern when in remission and when treatment has concluded, so that any final height deficiency is usually minimal (Swift et al., 1978; Shalet et al., 1979; Griffin and Wadsworth, 1980).

Although not necessarily endocrinal, various other somatic complications besides growth impairment and sterility have been reported following CNS prophylaxis for ALL. These include cardiopulmonary dysfunction, hepatic toxicity, renal toxicity and second malignancies (Meadows and Silber, 1985; Meadows and Hobbie, 1986; Meadows et al., 1989; Mulhern et al., 1989).

Cognitive changes

In addition to causing physical and endocrine abnormalities, many reports in the literature dating from the mid-1970s have indicated that CNS prophylaxis may also have detrimental effects on various cognitive functions. Cognition is the operation of the mind process by which we become aware of objects of thought and perception, including all aspects of perceiving, thinking and remembering. Thus, the term 'cognitive functioning' encompasses a range of abilities, including those traditionally assessed by a neuropsychologist, such as IQ, as well as personality, behaviour, attention, academic skills, and language abilities. Here, the term 'cognitive functions' is used to encompass these attributes. It is widely recognized that many cognitive and psychosocial adjustment problems are associated with paediatric chronic illness (Eiser, 1990; Madan-Swain and Brown, 1991). Often such problems stem directly from the disease itself. For instance, hypoglycaemia associated with diabetes mellitus has resulted in problems with school performance and concentration (Johnson, 1980);

similarly, cerebral vascular infarcts frequently associated with sickle cell disease lead to cognitive impairments in children (Fowler et al., 1976). On the other hand, other problems afflict all chronically ill children. For instance, school absence, lengthy hospitalizations and changes in family status — and these have been linked by some authors with cognitive and social problems. Madan-Swain and Brown (1991) have pointed out that such confounding factors render it extremely difficult to determine whether ALL itself directly affects cognitive functioning in children, and that researchers 'are faced with the dual task of examining the effects of a chronic illness as well as the unique effects of ALL and the treatments for it' (p. 268).

Intelligence

Amongst children receiving CNS prophylactic treatment (which may or may not include cranial irradiation) for ALL, several general cognitive effects have been reported. The most frequently tested parameter is IQ, usually involving administration of one of the Wechsler scales. Initial studies of survivors of ALL failed to demonstrate any permanent intellectual or behavioural impairment (Holmes and Holmes, 1975; Soni et al., 1975; Li and Stone, 1976; Verzosa et al., 1976). Indeed, certain later studies reported the same outcome (Berg et al., 1983; Inati et al., 1983; Mauer et al., 1983; Harten et al., 1984). However, other early studies did report problems, and amongst these studies, Eiser and Lansdown (1977) and Meadows et al. (1981) noticed particular IQ deficits in children who were younger at the time of CNS prophylaxis.

Brouwers et al. (1985) mentioned that more sophisticated studies reported significant functional defects, particularly in patients who were very young (aged less than four or five years) at the time of disease diagnosis (and therefore at the time of CNS prophylaxis).

Several researchers have reported the presence of intellectual impairment in children treated with cranial irradiation and chemotherapy for ALL (e.g. Eiser, 1978; Meadows et al., 1981; Duffner et al., 1985; Taylor et al., 1987). Some authors found IQ was lower than average compared with normative data (Eiser and Landsdown, 1977; Eiser, 1980; Meadows et al., 1981; Whitt et al., 1984; Copeland et al., 1985; Mulhern et al., 1987, 1988). Others found Full Scale IQ in children treated for ALL to be lower than their siblings or peers (Moss et al., 1981; Chessels, 1983, 1985; Jannoun, 1983; Twaddle et al., 1983, 1986; Said et al., 1987; Taylor et al., 1987; Schlieper et al., 1989; Brown et al., 1992). Yet other authors compared children who had received irradiation in other, non-CNS sites (e.g. for Wilms' tumour), and found that the ALL group performed more poorly on intelligence tests (Waber et al., 1990).

Large IQ deficits were noted by only two groups of investigators: Muchi et al. (1987), who recorded IQ scores of less than 80 in some subjects, and Mulhern et al. (1987), who examined relapsed ALL children and found mental retardation in 20% of them. Duffner et al. (1983) and Taylor et al. (1987) noted a subtle, but significant, lowering of intelligence quotients in long-term survivors of ALL.

Waber et al. (1990) assessed IQ [using the *Wechsler Intelligence Scale for Children — Revised* (WISC-R), Wechsler, 1974] and academic achievement (using the *Wide Range Achievement Test* (WRAT), Jastak and Jastak, 1978) in 51 children treated with cranial irradiation and IT MTX for ALL and 15 children treated with radiation and systemic chemotherapy for Wilms' tumour. The groups were compared with normative population data, and also with each other. Intra-group comparison to determine the effect of sex on neuropsychological parameters was also undertaken. The ALL group as a whole performed below the normative expectation. In particular, the scores of the female subjects on vocabulary, block design, arithmetic, digit span, coding, reading and spelling all fell below the test norms. The only scores that fell below the test norms for the males were the reading and spelling subtests of the WRAT.

In another leukaemia versus tumour study, Twaddle and colleagues (Twaddle et al., 1983) estimated the IQ level (from a corrected measure of sibling IQ) pre-treatment, for leukaemic and solid tumour patients who had been treated with a combination of MTX and cranial radiation (2400 rads). A difference in pre-treatment and post-treatment IQ was found in the ALL group, but not in the solid tumour group. Twaddle et al. (1983) noted that higher aspects of intelligence, such as verbal associate reasoning and reasoning with abstract material, were particularly vulnerable in the leukaemic group.

Performance IQ (as measured by the Wechsler scales) has been reported to be more affected than Verbal IQ (VIQ) by some authors (Eiser 1978, 1980; Meadows et al., 1981; Pfefferbaum-Levine et al., 1984; Brouwers et al., 1985; Copeland et al., 1985; Said et al., 1987). Copeland et al. (1985) noted that, within the performance subtests, the poorest scores occurred in visual–motor ability, spatial memory, fine motor ability, coding and arithmetic. However, apart from a study by Taylor et al. (1987), which included several language assessments amongst other cognitive assessments, most statements regarding the language abilities of post-treatment ALL subjects are based on global language measures such as VIQ scores, rather than specific linguistic assessments. Consequently, effects on language may have been missed owing to the lack of sufficiently sensitive or specifically designed measures of language.

Furthermore, Brouwers et al. (1984) pointed out a very important fact that has been largely overlooked by researchers supporting the Verbal–Performance discrepancy theory. The lower Performance IQ (PIQ) has been frequently thought to reflect a deficit in perceptuo–visual–spatial functioning. Kagan (1982), however, has drawn attention to the fact that the majority of subtests of which PIQ consists are timed tasks. Therefore, as argued by Brouwers et al. (1984), if ALL survivors demonstrated alterations in attention or functional slowing, PIQ would tend to decrease more than VIQ. Brouwers et al. (1984) found strong support for their reasoning when ALL survivors assessed did not demonstrate slowed reaction times.

A survey of 31 studies of cognitive functioning in children treated for ALL was conducted by Cousens et al. (1988). It was found that 16 out of the 31 publications demonstrated significant IQ deficits after CNS prophylaxis, seven reported non-significant or non-specific reductions, five yielded no effect, and the remaining three studies reported equivocal results. A meta-analysis was undertaken on 30 reported IQ patient–control comparisons in 20 different studies and found an average decrement in full score IQ of about 10 points (or 0.72 of a standard deviation).

Ochs and Mulhern (1988) stated that, despite the number of studies investigating the neuropsychological status of children treated for ALL that have been published (which amounted to more than 40 at the time of writing), specific conclusions have been hard to draw, as findings by authors have rarely been replicated, and methodological flaws exist in many studies. Nevertheless, in spite of the controversies regarding areas of deficit, studies have found some intellectual deficits in ALL survivors, and CNS prophylaxis (in the form of cranial irradiation or the combination of radiotherapy and IT MTX) is a primary factor implicated in the development of the reported mild neuropsychological deficits (Eiser, 1978; Tameroff et al., 1982; Tebbi, 1982; Jannoun, 1983; Ochs and Mulhern, 1988). Although an IQ deficit is well-documented, there is little understanding about the nature of the problems in cognitive functioning that may underly and result in the observed IQ deficits (Brouwers et al., 1984).

Despite the evidence that a combination of chemotherapy and radiotherapy in the form of CNS prophylaxis may have long-term effects on various neuropsychological abilities, the effect of chemotherapy alone on these functions is less certain. Tamaroff et al. (1982) failed to detect neuropsychological deficits following the administration of IT MTX. Forty-one children with ALL were assessed within one year of completing a 36-month course of IT MTX. MTX was administered at regular intervals in a dose of 6.25 mg/m^2 and was the sole agent of CNS prophylaxis. A control group of 33 children with embryonal rhabdomyosarcoma (ERMS) who had no central nervous disease or treatment were also studied. There was no significant difference in IQ between the two groups for children less than eight years of age. When children older than eight years were considered, those with ALL achieved IQ scores significantly greater than the children suffering from ERMS. In addition, 12 of the 21 younger children were reassessed at an average of 57.4 months after the initial examination. No long-term intellectual changes were detected. The authors concluded that IT MTX alone does not have either short-term or long-term effects on general intellectual functioning. Tamaroff et al. (1982) suggested that the 2400 rads of cranial radiation given to patients in other studies may be responsible for any reported deficits, or that perhaps radiation and MTX in combination produce the neurological deficits.

Language deficits

Considering the disruption to higher functions of intelligence outlined above, it could reasonably be expected that children treated for ALL would also demonstrate deficits in language function. To date, however, few studies have focused on the linguistic abilities of children treated for ALL. Higher-level language problems were identified by Taylor et al. (1987) in children with ALL post-irradiation. These researchers included four age-normed assessments of language (the *Expressive One Word Picture Vocabulary Test*, the *Token Test*, the *Word Fluency Test* and the *Verbal Selective Reminding Test*) in their test battery and reported that leukaemia subjects performed less well than their siblings on tasks requiring speed and accuracy (word fluency, contingency naming) and on a task requiring the ability to follow multiple element directions (the *Token Test*). Apart from the study by Taylor et al. (1987), however, the majority of comments in the literature relating to the language abilities of post-treatment ALL subjects are based on neuropsychological measures rather than on comprehensive language assessments. Consequently, although a number of authors have noted that language function remains intact following CNS prophylaxis in childhood leukaemia (Eiser, 1978, 1980; Brouwers et al., 1985; Copeland et al., 1985), effects on language may have been missed by these researchers due to the lack of sufficiently sensitive or specifically designed measures of language.

Buttsworth et al. (1993) and Murdoch et al. (1994) investigated the language abilities of a group of 22 children treated for ALL. They found that overall, the linguistic deficits exhibited by these children were mild. As a group, however, the leukaemia subjects performed significantly worse than age- and sex-matched control subjects on the *Test of Adolescent Language 2, Clinical Evaluation of Language Function* and *Boston Naming Test*. Individually, the leukaemia subjects varied in their performance on the language measures. The findings of Buttsworth et al. (1993) and Murdoch et al. (1994) are described and discussed in detail in Chapter 6.

Behaviour, attention and memory changes

A vital initial component of cognitive processing involves attention to stimuli operating in the outside environment (Brouwers et al., 1984).

The first mention of attention and behaviour problems in survivors of ALL was made by Meadows and Evans (1976), who, on the basis of informal observations, reported that most subjects with ALL demonstrated excessive inattentiveness and hyperactivity during the testing sessions.

A number of pertinent teacher rating studies also exist. For example, Verzosa et al. (1976) reported on teacher ratings of 22 children treated with irradiation for ALL, and found that one-third of their subjects were rated as below average in energy, motivation, attention span and abstract thinking. Similarly, in a study conducted by Cairns et al. (1980), teachers reported that nearly one-third of children surviving cancer demonstrated problems with attention and acting out. Teachers participating in a study by Deasy-Spinetta and Spinetta (1980) reported more attentional and learning problems in cancer survivors than in matched normal peers.

Later investigations of children treated for ALL have corroborated the presence of poor attention and concentration, distractibility, impulsivity and difficulty in processing information (e.g. Eiser, 1980; Goff et al., 1980; Pavlovsky et al., 1983; Brouwers et al., 1984; Pfefferbaum-Levine et al., 1984; Whitt, 1984; Chessells, 1985; Said et al., 1987, 1989). Brouwers et al. (1984) documented a strong correlation between the presence and type of CT scan abnormality in ALL children and attentional performance, such that ALL children with calcifications observed on their CT scans performed more poorly on attention tests than ALL children with evidence of cerebral atrophy.

Memory deficits in children treated for ALL are also frequently noted (Eiser, 1980; Goff et al., 1980; Meadows et al., 1981; Tamaroff et al., 1982; Brouwers et al., 1984; Pfefferbaum-Levine et al., 1984; Chessells, 1985; Copeland et al., 1985; Mulhern et al., 1988; Peckham et al., 1988; Said et al., 1989) and indeed are thought to play a vital role in observed intellectual and academic deficits. As Mulhern et al. (1988) pointed out, academic and intellectual impairments in ALL survivors have not been associated with an actual loss of previously acquired knowledge, and thus impairments observed are likely to be a result of a decreased rate of acquisition of new skills and information, due largely to memory problems (Meadows et al., 1981; Tamaroff et al., 1982; Brouwers et al., 1985; Mulhern et al., 1988).

Since Mulhern et al. (1988) considered memory to be a more sensitive indicator of learning aptitude than IQ or academic achievement, and a more appropriate gauge of impairment in ALL survivors, they administered a battery of memory tests to 40 ALL subjects on two different treatment protocols — with and without irradiation. No significant memory differences according to treatment, age at diagnosis or CT abnormalities were found. However, the ALL subjects were below normative expectation on verbal and visual–spatial memory abilities. Mulhern et al. (1988)

concluded that the deficit in memory ability could not be explained adequately by either irradiation, age at diagnosis, CT abnormalities, or lowered IQ, and subscribed to the idea that a factor common to all subjects, such as the disease itself or moderately aggressive systemic and/or intrathecal chemotherapy, may be responsible (Meadows and Evans, 1976; Invik et al., 1981).

The symptoms demonstrated by certain ALL children have been noted to bear a striking similarity to those exhibited by children with attention deficit disorder (ADD), also called attention deficit hyperactivity disorder (ADHD) (Cousens et al., 1990; Madan-Swain and Brown, 1991). However, it seems that not all characteristics are necessarily evident in all research. For instance, although Peckham et al. (1988) noted attention and concentration problems in ALL survivors, there was an absence of hyperactivity. Indeed, the subjects were generally less energetic than their peers. Conversely, Meadows and Evans (1976) found hyperactivity to be characteristic of ALL children during testing sessions.

Cousens et al. (1990) commented on a surprising resemblance between the cognitive deficit following CNS prophylaxis and that present in ADD. These authors compared ALL survivors with three other groups: children with solid tumours, children with ADD and ALL sibling control subjects on measures of memory, attention and aspects of cognitive functioning measured by Freedom from Distractibility from the WISC-R. Findings indicated that both the ALL group and the ADD group were significantly worse than the sibling control group on measures of distractibility, discrimination, memory and reaction time, with performance of the ADD group being consistently (and significantly) poorer than the ALL group. Cousens et al. (1990) interpreted these results to mean that the principal cognitive deficiencies of the ALL and ADD groups are on a continuum, with the ADD group typically performing at a lower level than the ALL group.

Academic achievement

Reports in the literature suggest that children treated for ALL exhibit deficits not only in IQ tests, but also on measures of academic achievement (Hallahan and Kauffman, 1978; Rowland et al., 1984; Whitt et al., 1984; Copeland et al., 1985; Moore, Kramer and Albin, 1986; Ochs et al., 1986; Taylor et al., 1987; Peckham et al., 1988; Madan-Swain and Brown, 1991). However, the actual relationship between CNS prophylaxis and academic problems is the subject of controversy and remains undefined (e.g. Lansky et al., 1984; Rowland et al., 1984; Williams and Davis, 1986; Mulhern et al., 1987, 1989), since academic problems may also be associated with school absences. Investigations involving teacher reports have also found progressive declines in academic achievement after ALL treatment (Cairns et al., 1980; Deasy-Spinetta and Spinetta, 1980).

The WRAT (Jastak and Jastak, 1978), which considers reading, spelling and arithmetic has been widely used to measure academic performances of ALL subjects and controls. Significantly poorer WRAT outcomes have been reported for leukaemic patients than for their siblings (e.g. Taylor et al., 1987) and solid tumour control subjects (e.g. Copeland et al., 1985; Moore et al., 1986). Peckham et al. (1988) suggested that visual and auditory memory problems in ALL survivors may have interfered with the acquisition of fundamental academic facts. Chessells (1985) similarly suggested that deficits in speed of information and auditory learning occur in children following CNS prophylaxis, but stressed that the hypothesis requires confirmation. Studies that have compared WRAT results of leukaemic patients who had received cranial irradiation, with those who had received prophylaxis consisting of drug therapy only, have not identified significant differences (Whitt et al., 1984; Copeland et al., 1985; Ochs et al., 1986).

Lansky et al. (1986) found that almost 30% of their sample of adult survivors of paediatric ALL reported having had academic problems at school. Similarly, Mulhern et al. (1989) found a similar rate of school problems in 183 ALL survivors.

Reading deficits have been found both in ALL children in complete continuous remission (Eiser, 1980; Said et al., 1989) and in children who have suffered a relapse (Mulhern et al., 1987). In addition, Mulhern et al. (1987) reported spelling and mathematical difficulties in children with ALL who had suffered a relapse.

Repeating grades and special education placement occur with relative frequency in children with ALL. For instance, Mulhern et al. (1989) surveyed 183 cancer survivors (of whom 45% had been ALL patients) and found that 26% had repeated one or more grades in school and 11% had a history of special education placement.

Eiser (1991) pointed out that academic achievement as measured by formal assessment may not reflect a child's true ability, and advocated that the reader take into account emotional possibilities. She wrote, 'Children's achievements in school are also dependent on intrapersonal factors such as self esteem and coping skills, as well as position in peer group' (p.167). Cousens et al. (1988) stated that children with leukaemia can experience lowered self-esteem and can be teased by peers. In a similar vein, school absence has been suggested by some authors to be a factor involved in academic problems in children with ALL. Lansky et al. (1984) found that, during the first year of treatment, leukaemic children miss an average of 42% of the school year, and moreover, there is also a substantial rate of absences in the second and third year.

Recent publications have drawn attention to the need to offer continuing support and remedial assistance to ALL survivors (Peckham et al., 1988; Mulhern et al., 1989) and have concluded that ALL survivors ought to be offered extra educational aid at school. The type of remedial assistance likely to provide the most benefit is a matter of debate (Eiser, 1991).

Visual and motor changes

Considerably less information exists regarding the integrity of visual and motor abilities in children subsequent to treatment for ALL. However, since various authors have briefly mentioned such problems, it ought to be included in a list of adverse sequelae of CNS prophylaxis for ALL.

Cousens et al. (1990) inferred a visual processing deficit in 43 ALL survivors, based on the proportion of tests they administered (on which the subjects performed poorly) that involved either a visuomotor or visual–perceptual component, together with cases where a particular skill deficit existed only in the visual modality. Studies of visual evoked potentials in ALL survivors have documented increased latencies (Russo et al., 1985; Muchi et al., 1987), although it is possible that optic nerve demyelination had occurred before the CNS prophylaxis and was due to a direct leukaemic disease effect (Hendin et al., 1974).

Motor deficits have also been reported in ALL survivors (e.g. McIntosh et al., 1976). Peckham et al. (1988) found that most ALL survivors were reported by teachers to exhibit problems with co-ordination in physical and sporting activities, and 'awkwardness' in gait. Handwriting problems in ALL survivors are frequently reported (Cousens et al., 1990).

Summary of adverse effects of chemotherapy

In summary, the cerebral and cerebellar changes reported to follow CNS chemotherapy vary between studies in terms of the sites and types of damage, and the clinical presentations described. Clinical symptoms ascribed to the administration of chemotherapy (in particular, MTX) have included disorientation to time and place, gait disturbance, impaired reading and arithmetical abilities (Pizzo et al., 1976), progressive flaccid paresis, mental deterioration (Skullerud and Halvorsen, 1978), spastic quadriplegia or paraplegia, aphasia, slurred speech and a depressed level of responsiveness (Meadows and Evans, 1976). The cerebral and cerebellar damage reported, in association with the aphasia and dysarthria noted by Meadows and Evans (1976), suggests that both speech and language deficits may occur when cytotoxic drugs (in particular MTX) have been administered to the CNS. Although some studies attribute the reported changes to MTX, two studies involved subjects who also received radiotherapy (Smith, 1975; Meadows and Evans,

1976). Isolating MTX as the sole cause of damage can be questioned in such cases. In addition, there are studies which failed to detect CNS changes in large groups of children who received chemotherapy but not radiotherapy (Ochs et al., 1980; Tamaroff et al., 1982). Such findings further question the validity of isolating MTX as the sole agent of damage when all or part of the subject group experienced irradiation in addition to the chemotherapy being examined.

Adverse effects of combined radiotherapy and chemotherapy

Overall, the CNS damage and deficits observed following combined radiotherapy and chemotherapy are similar to those reported when either treatment is administered alone and include focal lesions of the periventricular white matter, ventricular dilation, cortical atrophy, basal ganglia calcifications, widespread calcium deposits in the subcortical white and grey matter and in the cerebellar regions, demyelination, subcortical necrosis and cerebrovascular changes (Norrell et al., 1974; Arnold et al., 1978; Girault et al., 1978; Brouwers et al., 1985; Packer et al., 1986; Di Chiro et al., 1988).

Clinical manifestations of CNS prophylaxis have included:

- Akinetic mutism, expressive aphasia (Norrell et al., 1974).
- Language deficits (Kramer et al., 1988).
- Intellectual disabilities (Holmes and Holmes, 1975; Eiser, 1978; Meadows et al., 1981; Duffner et al., 1983; Brouwers et al., 1985; Kramer et al., 1988).
- Learning disabilities (Holmes and Holmes, 1975; Meadows et al., 1981; Moss et al., 1981; Duffner et al., 1983; Kramer et al., 1988).
- Ataxia and other physical disabilities (Holmes and Holmes, 1975; Duffner et al., 1983).

Whether the deficits associated with a combination of radiotherapy and chemotherapy are of greater severity than those observed when only one form of treatment is used has not been addressed.

Thus, the literature strongly suggests that children who receive any combination of radiotherapy and chemotherapy for CNS prophylactic treatment should be monitored closely for the appearance of CNS changes and/or declines in functional abilities.

References

Allen JC, Deck MDF, Howieson J, Brown M (1981) CT scans of long term survivors of various childhood malignancies. Medical Pediatric Oncology 9: 109–117.

Arnold H, Kuhne D, Franke H, Grosch I (1978) Finds in computerized axial tomography after intrathecal methotrexate and radiation. Neurology 16: 65–68.

Bamford FN, Morris-Jones P, Pearson D, Ribeiro GG, Shalet SM, Beardwell CG (1976) Residual disabilities in children treated for intracranial space-occupying lesions. Cancer 37: 1149–1151.

Bendersky M, Lewis M, Mandelbaum DE, Slanger C (1988) Serial neuropsychological follow-up of a child following craniospinal irradiation. Developmental Medicine and Child Neurology 30: 816–820.

Berg RA, Ch'ien LT, Bowman WP, Ochs J, Lancaster W, Goff JR, Anderson HR (1983) The neuropsychological effects of acute lymphocytic leukemia and its treatment — a three-year report: intellectual functioning and academic achievement. Clinical Neuropsychology 5: 9–13.

Bleyer WA, Griffin TW (1980) White matter necrosis, mineralizing microangiapathy, and intellectual abilities in survivors of childhood leukemia: associations with central nervous system irradiation and methotrexate therapy. In Gilbert HA, Kagan AR (eds) Radiation Damage to the Nervous System. New York: Raven: 155–174.

Brecher ML, Berger P, Freeman AI (1985) Computed tomographic scan findings in children with acute lymphoblastic leukemia treated with three different methods of CNS prophylaxis. Cancer 56: 2430–2433.

Broadbent VA, Barnes ND, Wheeler TK (1981) Medulloblastoma in childhood: long-term results of treatment. Cancer 48: 26–30.

Brouwers P, Riccardi R, Poplack D, Fedio P (1984) Attentional deficits in long-term survivors of childhood acute lymphoblastic leukemia (ALL). Journal of Clinical Neuropsychology 6: 325–336.

Brouwers P, Riccardi R, Fedio P, Poplack D (1985) Long-term neuropsychologic sequelae of childhood leukemia: correlation with CT brain scan abnormalities. Journal of Pediatrics 106: 723–728.

Brown RT, Madan-Swain A, Pais R, Lambert RG, Baldwin K, Casey R, Frank N, Sexson SB, Ragab A, Kamphaus RW (1992) Cognitive status of children treated with central nervous system prophylactic chemotherapy for acute lymphocytic leukemia. Archives of Clinical Neuropsychology 7: 481–497.

Buttsworth DL, Murdoch BE, Ozanne AE (1993) Acute lymphoblastic leukaemia: language deficits in children post-treatment. Disability and Rehabilitation 15: 67–75.

Cairns NU, Klopovich P, Moore R, Stephenson L, Fried P, Gradolf B, Suenram D, Kurz L, Butterfield G (1980) The dying child in the classroom. Essence 4: 25.

Cantini R, Giorgetti W, Valleriani AM, Burchianti M, Amodeo C (1989) Radiation-induced cerebral lesions in childhood. Child's Nervous System 5: 135–139.

Carli M, Perilongo G, Laverda AM, Drigo P, Casara GL, Marin G, Sotti G, Deambrosis G, Zanesco L (1985) Risk factors in long-term sequelae of central nervous system prophylaxis in successfully treated children with acute lymphocytic leukemia. Medical and Pediatric Oncology 13: 334–340.

Chessells JM (1983) Review: childhood acute lymphoblastic leukemia: the late effects of treatment. British Journal of Haematology 53: 369–378.

Chessells JM (1985) Cranial irradiation in childhood lymphoblastic leukaemia: time for reappraisal? British Medical Journal 291: 686.

Ch'ien LT, Rhomes JA, Verzosa MS, Coburn TP, Goff JR, Hustu HO, Price RA, Seifert MJ, Simone JV (1981) Progression of methotrexate-induced leukoencephalopathy in children with leukaemia. Medical and Pediatric Oncology 9: 133–141.

Chin HW, Maruyama Y (1984) Age at treatment and long-term performance results in medulloblastoma. Cancer 53: 1952–1958.

Civin CI (1989) Reducing the cost of the cure in childhood leukemia. New England Journal of Medicine 321: 185–187.

Copeland DR, Fletcher JM, Pfefferbaum-Levine B, Jaffe N, Reid H, Maor M (1985) Neuropsychological sequelae of childhood cancer in long-term survivors. Pediatrics 75: 745–753.

Cousens P, Waters JS, Said J, Stevens M (1988) Cognitive effects of cranial irradiation in leukemia: a survey and meta-analysis. Journal of Child Psychology and Psychiatry 29: 938–952.

Cousens P, Ungerer JA, Crawford JA, Stevens MM (1990) The nature and possible causes of cognitive deficit after childhood leukemia. Brain Impairment: Advances in Applied Research: Proceedings of the Fifteenth Annual Conference of the Australian Society for the Study of Brain Impairment: 173–181.

Crosley CJ, Rourke LB, Evans A, Nigro M (1978) Central nervous system lesions in childhood leukemia. Neurology 28: 678–685.

Curnes JT, Laster DW, Ball MR, Moody DM, Witcofski RL (1986) MRI of radiation injury to the brain. American Journal of Roentgenology 147: 119–124.

Danoff BF, Chowchock FS, Marquette C, Mulgrew L, Kramer S (1982) Assessment of the long-term effects of primary radiation therapy for brain tumours in children. Cancer 49: 1580–1586.

Davis PC, Hoffman JC, Pearl GS, Braun IF (1986) CT evaluation of effects of cranial radiation therapy in children. American Journal of Roentgenology 147: 587–592.

Day RE, Kingston J, Bullimore JA, Mott MG, Thomson JLG (1978) CAT brain scans after central nervous system prophylaxis for acute lymphoblastic leukaemia. British Medical Journal 2: 1752–1753.

Deasy-Spinetta P, Spinetta J (1980) The child with cancer in school. American Journal of Pediatric Hematology–Oncology 2: 89.

De Reuck J, vander Eecken H (1975) The anatomy of the late radiation encephalopathy. European Neurology 13: 481–494.

Deutsch M (1982) Radiotherapy for primary brain tumours in very young children. Cancer 50: 2785–2789.

Di Chiro G, Oldfield W, Wright DC, De Michele D, Katz DA, Patronas NJ, Doppman JL, Larson SM, Ito M, Kufta CV (1988) Cerebral necrosis after radiotherapy and/or intraarterial chemotherapy for brain tumours: PET and neuropathological studies. American Journal of Roentgenology 150: 189–197.

Di Lorenzo N, Nolletti A, Palma L (1978) Late cerebral radionecrosis. Surgical Neurology 10: 281–290.

Dooms GC, Hecht S, Brant-Zawadzki M, Berthiaume Y, Norman D, Newton TH (1986) Brain radiation lesions: MR imaging. Radiology 158: 149–155.

Duffner PK, Cohen ME, Thomas PRM (1983) Late effects of treatment on the intelligence of children with posterior fossa tumours. Cancer 51: 233–237.

Duffner PK, Cohen ME, Thomas RM, Lansky SB (1985) The long-term effects of cranial irradiation on the central nervous system. Cancer 56: 1841–1846.

Eiser C (1978) Intellectual abilities among survivors of childhood leukaemia as a function of CNS irradiation. Archives of Disease in Childhood 53: 391–395.

Eiser C (1980) Effects of chronic illness on intellectual development: a comparison of normal children with those treated for childhood leukaemia and solid tumours. Archives of Disease in Childhood 55: 766–770.

Eiser C (1990) Chronic Childhood Disease. Cambridge: Cambridge University.

Eiser C (1991) Cognitive deficits in children treated for leukaemia. Archives of Disease in Childhood 66: 164–168.

Eiser C, Lansdown R (1977) Retrospective study of intellectual development in children treated for acute lymphoblastic leukaemia. Archives of Disease in Childhood 52: 525–529.

Enzmann DR, Lane B (1978) Enlargement of subarachnoid spaces and lateral ventricles in pediatric patients undergoing chemotherapy. Journal of Pediatrics 92: 535–539.

Esseltine DW, Freeman CR, Chevalier LM, Smith R, O'Gorman AM, Dube J, Whitehead VM, Nogrady MB (1981) Computed tomography brain scans in long term survivors of childhood acute lymphoblastic leukemia. Medical Pediatric Oncology 9: 429–438.

Fletcher JM, Copeland DR (1988) Neurobehavioral effects of central nervous system prophylactic treatment of cancer in children. Journal of Clinical and Experimental Neuropsychology 10: 495–538.

Fossati-Bellani F, Gasparini M, Lombardi F, Zucali R, Luccarelli G, Migliavacca F, Moise S, Nicola G (1984) Medulloblastoma: results of a sequential combined treatment. Cancer 54: 1956–1961.

Fowler J, Budzynski T, Vandenbergh R (1976) Effects of an EMG biofeedback program on the control of diabetes: a case study. Biofeedback and Self-regulation 1: 105–112.

Freeman JE, Johnston PGB, Voke JM (1973) Somnolence after prophylactic cranial irradiation in children with acute lymphoblastic leukaemia. British Medical Journal 4: 523–525.

Giralt M, Gil JL, Borderas F, Oliveros A, Gomez-Pereda R, Pardo J, Martinez-Ibanez F, Raichs A (1978) Intracerebral calcifications in childhood lymphoblastic leukemia. Acta Haematologica 59: 193–204.

Goff JR, Anderson HR, Cooper PF (1980) Distractibility and memory deficits in long-term survivors of acute lymphoblastic leukemia. Journal of Developmental and Behavioral Pediatrics 1: 158–163.

Griffin NK, Wadsworth J (1980) Effects of treatment of malignant disease on growth in children. Archives of Disease in Childhood 55: 600–603.

Habermalz E, Habermalz HJ, Stephani U, Henze G, Riehm H, Hanefeld F (1983) Cranial computed tomography of 64 children in continuous complete remission of leukemia I: Relations to therapy modalities. Neuropediatrics 14: 144–148.

Hallahan DP, Kauffman JM (1978) Exceptional Children: Introduction to Special Education. Englewood Cliffs, NJ: Prentice-Hall.

Harten G, Stephani U, Henze G, Langermann HJ, Riehm H, Hanefeld F (1984) Slight impairment of psychomotor skills in children after treatment of acute lymphoblastic leukemia. European Journal of Pediatrics 142: 189–197.

Hendin B, De Vivo DC, Torak R, Lell ME, Ragab AH, Vietti TJ (1974) Parenchymatous degeneration of the central nervous system in childhood leukemia. Cancer 33: 468–482.

Holmes HA, Holmes FF (1975) After ten years, what are the handicaps and lifestyles of children treated for cancer? An examination of the present status of 124 survivors. Clinical Pediatrics 14: 819–823.

Hoppe-Hirsch E, Renier D, Lellouch-Tubiana A, Sainte-Rose C, Pierre-Kahn A, Hirsch JF (1990) Medulloblastoma in childhood: progressive intellectual deterioration. Child's Nervous System 6: 60–65.

Hudson LJ, Murdoch BE (1992a) Language recovery following surgery and CNS prophylaxis for the treatment of childhood medulloblastoma: a prospective study of three cases. Aphasiology 6: 17–28.

Hudson LJ, Murdoch BE (1992b) Chronic language deficits in children treated for posterior fossa tumour. Aphasiology 6: 135–150.

Hudson LJ, Murdoch BE, Ozanne AE (1989) Posterior fossa tumours in childhood: associated speech and language disorders post-surgery. Aphasiology 3: 1–18.

Inati A, Sallan SE, Cassidy RJ, Hitchock-Bryan S, Clavell LA, Belli JA, Sollee N (1983) Efficacy and morbidity of central nervous system 'prophylaxis' in childhood acute lymphoblastic leukemia: eight years' experience with cranial irradiation and intrathecal methotrexate. Blood 61: 297–303.

Invik RJ, Colligan RC, Obetz SW, Smithson WA (1981) Neuropsychologic performance among children in remission from acute lymphocytic leukemia. Journal of Developmental and Behavioural Pediatrics 2: 29–34.

Jannoun L (1983) Are cognitive and educational development affected by age at which prophylactic therapy is given in acute lymphoblastic leukaemia? Archives of Disease in Childhood 58: 953–958.

Jastak JF, Jastak S (1978) Wide Range Achievement Test. Revised edition. Wilmington, DE: Jastak.

Johnson SB (1980) Psychosocial factors in juvenile diabetics: a review. Journal of Behavioral Medicine 3: 95–116.

Kagan J (1982) The idea of spatial ability. New England Journal of Medicine 306: 1225–1227.

Kearsley JH (1983) Late cerebrovascular disease after radiation therapy — report of two cases and a review of the literature. Australasian Radiology 27: 11–18.

Kirk JA, Stevens M, Menser MA, Tink A, Raghupathy P, Cowell CT, Bergin M, Vines RH, Silink M (1987) Growth failure and growth-hormone deficiency after treatment for acute lymphoblastic leukaemia. Lancet i: 190–193.

Kolmannskogg S, Moe PJ, Anke IM (1979) Computed tomographic findings of the brain in children with acute lymphocytic leukaemia after central nervous system prophylaxis without cranial irradiation. Acta Paediatrica Scandinavica 68: 875–877.

Kramer JH, Norman D, Brant-Zawadzki M, Ablin A, Moore IM (1988) Absence of white matter changes on magnetic resonance imaging in children treated with CNS prophylaxis therapy for leukaemia. Cancer 61: 928–930.

Kun LE, Mulhern RK, Crisco JJ (1983) Quality of life in children treated for brain tumours. Journal of Neurosurgery 58: 1–6.

Lansky SB, Cairns NU, Lansky LL, Cairns GF, Stephenson L, Garin G (1984) Central nervous system prophylaxis: studies showing impairment in verbal skills and academic achievement. American Journal of Pediatric Hematology/Oncology 6: 183–190.

Lansky SB, List MA, Ritter-Sterr C (1986) Psychological consequences of cure. Cancer 58: 529–533.

LeBaron S, Zeltzer PM, Zeltzer LK, Scott SE, Marlin AE (1988) Assessment of quality of survival in children with medulloblastoma and cerebellar astrocytoma. Cancer 62: 1215–1222.

Lee KF, Suh JH (1977) CT evidence of grey matter calcification secondary to radiation therapy. Computerized Tomography 1: 103–110.

Li FP, Stone R (1976) Survivors of cancer in childhood. Annals of International Medicine 84: 551–553.

Lichtor T, Wollman RL, Brown FD (1984) Calcified basal ganglionic mass 12 years after radiation therapy for medulloblastoma. Surgical Neurology 21: 373–376.

Madan-Swain A, Brown RT (1991) Cognitive and psychological sequelae for children with acute lymphocytic leukemia and their families. Clinical Psychology Review 11: 267–294.

Marks JE, Baglan RJ, Prassad SC, Blank WF (1981) Cerebral radionecrosis: incidence and risk in relation to dose, time, fractionation and volume. International Journal of Radiation Oncology, Biology and Physics 7: 243–252.

Martins AN, Johnston JS, Henry JM, Stoffel TJ, Di Chiro G (1977) Delayed radiation necrosis of the brain. Journal of Neurosurgery 47: 336–345.

Mauer AM, Ochs WP, Bowman L, Ch'ien W, Evans W, Ragland R, Parvey L, Coburn T, Simone JV (1983) Central nervous system prophylaxis for therapy of acute lymphocytic leukemia. In Mastrangelo R, Poplack DG, Riccardi R (eds) Central Nervous System Leukemia. Boston, MA: Martinus Nijhoff: 37–51.

McIntosh S, Lkatskin EH, O'Brien RT, Aspnes GT, Kammerer BL, Snead C, Kalavsky SM, Pearson HA (1976) Chronic neurologic disturbance in childhood leukemia. Cancer 37: 853–857.

McIntosh S, Fisher D, Rothman S, Rosenfield N, Lobel JS, O'Brien RT (1977) Intracranial calcifications in childhood leukemia. Journal of Pediatrics 91: 909–913.

Meadows AT, Evans AE (1976) Effects of chemotherapy on the central nervous system. Cancer 37: 1079–1085.

Meadows AT, Silber J (1985) Delayed consequences of therapy for childhood cancer. CA — A Cancer Journal for Clinicians 35: 271–286.

Meadows AT, Hobbie WL (1986) The medical consequences of cure. Cancer 58: 524–528.

Meadows AT, Massari DJ, Ferguson J, Gordon J, Littman P, Moss K (1981). Declines in IQ scores and cognitive dysfunctions in children with acute lymphocytic leukaemia treated with cranial irradiation. Lancet ii: 1015–1018.

Meadows AT, Robison LL, Sather H (1989) Potential long-term toxic effects in children treated for acute lymphoblastic leukemia [Letter to the Editor]. New England Journal of Medicine 321: 1830.

Moore IA, Kramer J, Albin A (1986) Late effects of central nervous system prophylactic leukaemia treatment on cognitive functioning. Oncology Nursing Forum 13: 45–51.

Moss HA, Nannis ED, Poplack DG (1981) The effects of prophylactic treatment of the central nervous system on the intellectual functioning of children with acute lymphoblastic leukemia. American Journal of Medicine 71: 47–52.

Muchi H, Satoh T, Kayoko Y, Karube T, Miyao M (1987) Studies on the assessment of neurotoxicity in children with acute lymphoblastic leukemia. Cancer 59: 891–895.

Mulhern RK, Williams JM, Le Sure SS, Kun LE (1986) Neuropsychological performance of children surviving cerebellar tumours: six case studies. Clinical Neuropsychology 8: 72–76.

Mulhern RK, Ochs J, Fairclough D, Wasserman AL, Davis KS, Williams JM (1987) Intellectual and academic achievement status after CNS relapse: a retrospective analysis of 40 children treated for acute lymphoblastic leukemia. Journal of Clinical Oncology 5: 933–940.

Mulhern RK, Wasserman AL, Fairclough D, Ochs J (1988) Memory function in disease-free survivors of childhood acute lymphocytic leukemia given central nervous system prophylaxis with or without 1800 cGy cranial irradiation. Journal of Clinical Oncology 6: 315–320.

Mulhern RK, Wasserman AL, Friedman AG, Fairclough D (1989) Social competence and behavioral adjustment of children who are long-term survivors of cancer. Pediatrics 83: 18–25.

Murdoch BE, Hudson-Tennent LJ (1994a) Differential language outcomes in children following treatment for posterior fossa tumours. Aphasiology 8: 507–534.

Murdoch BE, Hudson-Tennent LJ (1994b) Speech disorders in children treated for posterior fossa tumours. European Journal of Disorders of Communication 29: 379–397.

Murdoch BE, Boon DL, Ozanne AE (1994) Variability of language outcomes in children treated for acute lymphoblastic leukaemia: an examination of 23 cases. Journal of Medical Speech–Language Pathology 2: 113–123.

Nightingale S, Dawes PJDK, Cartlidge NEF (1982) Early-delayed radiation rhomben-
    cephalopathy. Journal of Neurology, Neurosurgery, and Psychiatry 45: 267–270.
Norrell H, Wilson CB, Slagel DE, Clark DB (1974) Leukoencephalopathy following
    the administration of methotrexate into the cerebrospinal fluid in the treatment
    of primary brain tumours. Cancer 33: 923–932.
Obetz S, Smithson W, Groover R, Houser O, Klass D, Ivnik R, Colligan R, Gilchrist G,
    Burgert E (1979) Neuropsychologic follow-up study of children with acute lym-
    phocytic leukemia. American Journal of Pediatric Hematology and Oncology 1:
    207–213.
Ochs JJ, Mulhern RK (1988) Late effects of antileukemic treatment. Pediatric Clinics of
    North America 35: 815–833.
Ochs JJ, Berger P, Brecher ML, Sinks LF, Kinkel W, Freeman AI (1980) Computed
    tomography brain scans in children with acute lymphoblastic leukemia receiving
    methotrexate alone as central nervous system prophylaxis. Cancer 45:
    2274–2278.
Ochs JJ, Parvey LS, Whitaker JN, Bowman WP, Ch'ien L, Campbell M, Coburn T (1983)
    Serial cranial computed tomography scans in children with leukemia given two
    different forms of central nervous system therapy. Journal of Clinical Oncology 1:
    793–798.
Ochs JJ, Parvey LS, Mulhern R (1986) Prospective study of central nervous system
    changes in children with acute lymphoblastic leukaemia receiving two different
    methods of central nervous system prophylaxis. Neurotoxicology 7: 217–226.
Packer RJ, Zimmerman RA, Bilaniuk LT (1986) Magnetic resonance imaging in the eval-
    uation of treatment-related central nervous system damage. Cancer 58: 635–640.
Packer RJ, Sutton LN, Atkins TE, Radcliffe J, Bunin GR, D'Angio G, Siegel KR, Schut L
    (1989) A prospective study of cognitive function in children receiving whole-brain
    radiotherapy and chemotherapy: 2-year results. Journal of Neurosurgery 70:
    707–713.
Painter MJ, Chutorian AM, Hilal SK (1975) Cerebrovasculopathy following irradiation
    in childhood. Neurology 25: 189–194.
Paolucci G, Rosito P (1983) Adverse sequelae of central nervous system prophylaxis
    in acute lymphoblastic leukemia. In Mastrangelo R, Poplack DR, Riccardi R (eds)
    Central Nervous System Leukemia. Boston, MA: Martinus Nijhoff: 105–112.
Pavlovsky S, Eastano J, Lerguardo R, Fisman N, Chamoles N, Moreno R, Aarizago R
    (1983) Neuropsychological study in patients with ALL. American Journal of
    Pediatric Hematology/Oncology 5: 78–86.
Pearson ADJ, Campbell AN, McAllister VL, Pearson GL (1983) Intracranial calcification
    in survivors of childhood medulloblastoma. Archives of Disease in Childhood 58:
    133–136.
Peckham VC, Meadows AT, Bartel N, Marrero O (1988) Educational late effects in
    long-term survivors of childhood acute lymphocytic leukemia. Pediatrics 81:
    127–133.
Peylan-Ramu N, Poplack DG, Pizzo PA, Adornato BT, Di Chiro G (1978) Abnormal CT
    scans in asymptomatic children with acute lymphocytic leukaemia after prophy-
    lactic treatment of the central nervous system with radiation and intrathecal
    chemotherapy. New England Journal of Medicine 298: 815–818.
Pfefferbaum-Levine B, Copeland DR, Fletcher JM, Ried HL, Jaffe N, McKinnon WR
    (1984) Neuropsychological assessment of long-term survivors of childhood
    leukemia. American Journal of Pediatric Hematology/Oncology 6: 123–128.
Pizzo PA, Bleyer WA, Poplack DG, Leventhal BG (1976) Reversible dementia tempo-
    rally associated with intraventricular therapy with methotrexate in a child with
    acute myelogenous leukaemia. Journal of Pediatrics 88: 131–133.

Pizzo PA, Poplack DG, Bleyer WA (1979) Neurotoxicities of current leukaemia therapy. American Journal of Paediatric Hematology and Oncology 1: 127–140.

Poplack DG (1983). Evaluation of adverse sequelae of central nervous system prophylaxis in acute lymphoblastic leukemia. In Mastrangelo R, Poplack DG, Riccardi R
(eds) Central Nervous System Leukemia. Boston, MA: Martinus Nijhoff: 95–103.

Price DB, Hotson GC, Loh JP (1988) Pontine calcification following radiotherapy: CT
demonstration. Journal of Computed Assisted Tomography 12: 45–46.

Price RA, Jamieson PA (1975) The central nervous system in childhood leukemia: II.
Subacute leukoencephalopathy. Cancer 35: 306–318.

Price RA, Birdwell DA (1978) The central nervous system in childhood leukaemia: III.
Mineralizing microangropathy and dystrophic calcification. Cancer 42: 717–728.

Riccardi R, Brouwers P, Di Chiro G, Poplack D (1985) Abnormal computed tomography brain scans in children with acute lymphoblastic leukemia: serial long-term
follow-up. Journal of Clinical Oncology 3: 12–18.

Riva D, Pantaleoni C, Milani N, Fossati-Belani F (1989) Impairment of neuropsychological functions in children with medulloblastomas and astrocytomas in the posterior fossa. Child's Nervous System 5: 107–110.

Rivera-Luna R, Rueda-Franco F, Lanche-Guevara MT, Martinez-Buerra G (1987)
Multidisciplinary treatment of medulloblastomas in childhood. Child's Nervous
System 3: 228–231.

Rowland JH, Glidewell OJ, Sibley RF, Holland JC, Tull R, Berman A, Brecher MI,
Harris M, Glicksman AS, Forman E, Jones B, Cohen ME, Duffner PE, Freeman AJ
(1984). Effects of different forms of central nervous system prophylaxis on neuropsychological function in childhood leukemia. Journal of Clinical Oncology 2:
1327–1335.

Russo A, Tomarchio S, Pero G, Consoli G, Marina R, Rizzari C, Schiliro G (1985)
Abnormal visual-evoked potentials in leukemic children after cranial radiation.
Medical and Pediatric Oncology 13: 313–317.

Said JA, Waters BGH, Cousens P, Stevens MM (1987) Neuropsychological after-effects
of central nervous system prophylaxis in survivors of childhood acute lymphoblastic leukaemia. In Gates GR (ed.) Proceeding of the Twelfth Annual Brain
Impairment Conference. Armidale: Australian Society for the Study of Brain
Impairment.

Said JA, Waters BGH, Cousens P, Stevens MM (1989) Neuropsychological sequelae of
central nervous system prophylaxis in survivors of childhood acute lymphoblastic
leukemia. Journal of Consulting and Clinical Psychology 57: 251–256.

Sainsbury CPQ, Newcombe RG, Hughes IA (1985) Weight gain and height velocity
during prolonged first remission from acute lymphoblastic leukemia. Archives of
Disease in Childhood 60: 832–836.

Schlieper AE, Esseltine DW, Tarshis E (1989) Cognitive function in long survivors of
childhood acute lymphoblastic leukemia. Pediatric Hematology and Oncology 6:
1–9.

Shalet SM, Price DA, Beardwell CG, Morris Jones PH, Pearson D (1979) Normal
growth despite abnormalities of growth hormone secretion in children treated
for acute leukemia. Journal of Pediatrics 94: 719–722.

Silverman CL, Palkes H, Talent B, Kovnar E, Clouse JW, Thomas PRM (1984) Late
effects of radiotherapy on patients with cerebellar medulloblastoma. Cancer 54:
825–829.

Skullerud L, Halvorsen L (1978) Encephalomyelopathy following intrathecal
methotrexate treatment in a child with acute leukaemia. Cancer 42: 1211–1215.

Smith B (1975) Brain damage after intrathecal methotrexate. Journal of Neurology,
Neurosurgery and Psychiatry 38: 810–815.

Soni SS, Marten GW, Pitner SE, Duenas DA, Powazek M (1975) Effects of central-nervous-system irradiation of neuropsychologic functioning of children with acute lymphocytic leukemia. New England Journal of Medicine 293: 113–117.

Swift PGK, Kearney PJ, Dalton RG, Bullimore JA, Mott MG, Savage DCL (1978) Growth and hormonal status of children treated for acute lymphoblastic leukaemia. Archives of Disease in Childhood 53: 890–894.

Tamaroff M, Miller DR, Murphy ML, Salwen R, Ghavimi R, Nir Y (1982) Immediate and long-term post-therapy neuropsychologic performance in children with acute lymphoblastic leukemia treated without central nervous system radiation. Journal of Pediatrics 101: 524–529.

Taylor HG, Albo VC, Phebus CK, Sachs BR, Bierl PG (1987) Postirradiation treatment outcomes for children with acute lymphocytic leukaemia: clarification of risks. Journal of Pediatric Psychology 12: 395–411.

Tebbi CK (1982) Major Topics in Pediatric and Adolescent Oncology. Boston, MA: GK Hall Medical Publishers.

Tsuruda JS, Kortman KE, Bradley WG, Wheeler DC, Van Dalsem W, Bradley TP (1987) Radiation effects on cerebral white matter: MR evaluation. American Journal of Roentgenology 149: 165–171.

Twaddle V, Britton PG, Craft AC, Noble TC, Kernahan J (1983) Intellectual function after treatment for leukaemia or solid tumours. Archives of Disease in Childhood 58: 949–952.

Twaddle V, Britton PG, Kernahan J, Craft AC (1986) Intellect after malignancy. Archives of Disease in Childhood 61: 700–702.

Verzosa M, Aur R, Simone J, Hustu H, Pinkel D (1976) Five years after central nervous system irradiation of children with leukemia. International Journal of Radiation Oncology, Biology, and Physics 1: 209–215.

Waber DP, Gioia G, Paccia J, Sherman B, Dinklage D, Sollee N, Tarbell NJ, Sallen SE (1990) Sex differences in cognitive processing in children treated with CNS prophylaxis for acute lymphoblastic leukemia (ALL). Journal of Pediatric Psychology 15: 105–122.

Wechsler D (1974) Manual for the Wechsler Intelligence Scale for Children. Revised. New York: Psychological Corporation.

Whitt JK, Wells RJ, Lauria MM, Wilhem CL, McMillan CW (1984) Cranial radiation in childhood acute lymphocytic leukemia: neuropsychologic sequelae. American Journal of Disease in Childhood 138: 730–736.

Williams JH, Davis KS (1986) Neuropsychological effects of central nervous system prophylactic treatment for childhood leukemia. Cancer Treatment Review 13: 113–127.

Wright TL, Bresnan MJ (1976) Radiation induced cerebrovascular disease in children. Neurology 26: 540–543.

Yamashita J, Handa H, Yumitori K, Abe M (1980) Reversible delayed radiation effect on the brain after radiotherapy of malignant astrocytoma. Surgical Neurology 13: 413–417.

Zurlo MG, Senesi E, Terranni B, Balducci D, Biddau P, D'Angelo P, Rosati D, Gandus S, Madon E, Mancini A, Nespoli L, Paicentini P, Veronesi SR, Tamato P (1988) Height of children off therapy after acute lymphoblastic leukemia. Pediatric Hematology and Oncology 5: 187–195.

Chapter 3
Language disorders in children treated for brain tumours

BRUCE E MURDOCH AND LISA J HUDSON

Introduction

Acquired language disorders are a recognized sequelae of treatment for brain tumours in childhood (Bamford et al., 1976; Danoff et al., 1982; Hudson et al., 1989; Hudson and Murdoch, 1992; Murdoch and Hudson-Tennent, 1994). As indicated in Chapter 1, tumours located in the posterior cranial fossa (i.e. infratentorial tumours involving the cerebellum, fourth ventricle and/or brainstem) occur more commonly in childhood than supratentorial neoplasms. In fact, up to 70% of all paediatric intracranial neoplasms occur in the posterior cranial fossa (Segall et al., 1985; Kadota et al., 1989; Russell and Rubinstein, 1989). Given the high prevalence of posterior fossa tumours in childhood, the present chapter will focus primarily on language disturbances reported in association with brain tumours involving the cerebellum, fourth ventricle and/or brainstem.

The location of the majority of childhood brain tumours in the posterior cranial fossa does not lead to the prediction of an associated language deficit. Despite this, there are a number of factors occurring secondary to the presence and removal of posterior fossa tumours that could conceivably lead to disturbances in language function. For example, in that they emerge from or invade the fourth ventricle, thereby obstructing the flow of cerebrospinal fluid, posterior fossa tumours are frequently accompanied by hydrocephalus. Compression of the cerebral cortex due to dilation of the ventricular system associated with hydrocephalus could conceivably impair the language abilities of these children. The mass effect of the tumour itself may also impede the flow of cerebrospinal fluid as well as contribute to tissue destruction and cortical compression. The invasion and compression of cerebral tissue may also result in vascular changes which could be related to the dysfunction in the central speech and language centres. In addition, radiotherapy, often given after surgical removal of certain types of posterior fossa tumours in order to prevent tumour spread or recurrence, has been reported to cause aphasia in some adults and intellectual deficits in some children (Broadbent et al., 1981; Danoff et al., 1982; Duffner et al., 1983; Kun et al., 1983; Burns and Boyle, 1984; Silverman et al., 1984). It is noteworthy, however, that any language deficits associated with radiotherapy may only appear in the long term, as the negative effects of radiotherapy have been reported to appear as delayed reactions (Hodges and Smithells, 1983; Pearson et al., 1983).

Despite posterior fossa tumours being the most common type of paediatric intracranial neoplasm and the existence of a number of factors occurring secondary to the removal of these tumours that could conceivably disturb language function, few studies have systematically investigated the language abilities of children treated for posterior fossa tumours. The majority of studies reported to date that have investigated acquired childhood language disorders have only included tumour cases in larger samples that also include children with acquired language disorders of differing aetiologies (Alajouanine and Lhermitte, 1965; Hécaen, 1976; Carrow-Woolfolk and Lynch, 1982; Miller et al., 1984; Van Dongen et al., 1985; Cooper and Flowers, 1987). In particular, these latter studies did not differentiate between various causes of acquired childhood language disorders, nor do they describe tumour sites or treatments. The most detailed studies of the language abilities of children treated for posterior fossa tumours to date are those reported by Hudson, Murdoch and colleagues (Hudson et al., 1989; Hudson and Murdoch, 1992; Murdoch and Hudson-Tennent, 1994). Consequently, this chapter will focus on providing a synthesis of their findings.

Language disorders and posterior fossa tumours

Evidence from mixed aetiology studies

Documentation of disturbances in the language function of children treated for brain tumours has appeared in reports of studies of acquired aphasia involving children with a variety of different aetiological conditions, including traumatic brain injury, cerebrovascular accidents and epilepsy among others. Two children who had undergone surgery for astrocytoma removal were included among 32 children with cerebral lesions studies by Alajouanine and Lhermitte (1965). As the sites of the tumours were not reported it cannot be confirmed whether the tumours were located in the posterior cranial fossa. Although as stated earlier, a posterior fossa location is more common in children, astrocytomas can also originate in the cerebral hemispheres.

The most prominent feature of the acquired language disorders exhibited by the subject group examined by Alajouanine and Lhermitte (1965), was a reduction of expressive activities (oral, written and gestures), a feature noted in all 32 children and not related to the presence of dysarthria. Two other studies involving tumour subjects have also reported a reduction of oral expression (Rekate et al., 1985; Volcan et al., 1986). The reduction of expression noted in these latter two studies, however, may have been caused by the presence of mutism and/or dysarthria rather than representing a disturbance in language function. Alajouanine and Lhermitte (1965) also noted the presence of severe reading and writing disturbances. Syntax was noted to be simplified rather than erroneous. Characteristics of aphasia seen in adults such as logorrhea, phonemic or semantic paraphasias, verbal stereotypes and perseverations, however, were not detected. The general pattern of simplified syntax, severe reading and writing disturbances and reduced oral expression is commonly reported in the literature with comprehension and word-finding difficulties also being exhibited by some children with acquired language disorders (Satz and Bullard-Bates, 1981; Carrow-Woolfolk and Lynch, 1982; Van Dongen et al., 1985).

Cooper and Flowers (1987) used a battery of language and academic tests to assess the language abilities of 15 children with histories of closed head injury (CHI), stroke, encephalitis or brain tumour (computerized tomography (CT) showed evidence of a posterior fossa mass in one child). As a group these subjects performed at a level significantly below that of a group of non-brain-injured control subjects in the areas of word, sentence and paragraph comprehension, naming, oral production of complex syntactic constructions and word fluency. Within the subject group, however, language deficits ranged from no or mild impairments to significant language deficits. Of particular interest was that the child who had been treated for posterior fossa tumour when 10 years old, had, when six years old, demonstrated aphasia, reduced receptive language skills and monosyllabic verbalizations at the time of diagnosis. Twelve months later, the same child was enrolled in full-time special education and was receiving speech therapy, occupational therapy and physiotherapy. On assessment, particular difficulties were noted on sentence formulation and naming tasks. Unfortunately, details of the medical management of this case were not provided. Hécaen (1976) also included two children with brain tumours in his study of 26 children with cortical lesions. He reported that in one of these two cases, the presence of a tumour in the left cerebral hemisphere resulted in muteness lasting two months, and articulation, reading and writing disorders from which there was no change.

Evidence from posterior fossa tumour case studies

Hudson et al. (1989) were the first authors to systematically examine the language abilities of children treated for posterior fossa tumours by use of a battery of specific language tests. They examined six children who had undergone surgery for removal of a posterior fossa tumour at least

12 months prior to language assessment. All six subjects examined had a negative history of birth trauma, head trauma, intellectual handicap, pre-morbid speech and/or language deficit or other neurological disorder and were monolingual speakers of English. Depending on their age at the time of testing, each of the six tumour cases reported by Hudson et al. (1989), were given one of the following three language tests:

- *Test of Language Development — Primary* (TOLD-P) (Newcomer and Hammill, 1982).
- *Test of Language Development — Intermediate* (TOLD-I) (Hammill and Newcomer, 1982).
- *Test of Adolescent Language 2* (TOAL-2) (Hammill et al., 1987).

In addition, each subject was also given Subtests 7 (Producing Word Series), 8 (Producing Names on Confrontation) and 9 (Producing Word Associations) of the *Clinical Evaluation of Language Functions* (CELF) (Semel and Wiig, 1982). The subjects showed language abilities that ranged from normal to severely impaired, a language impairment being evidenced in four of the six children studied. It was noted that the four children with evidence of language deficits had received central nervous system (CNS) prophylaxis (see Chapter 2) after surgery, whereas the two cases with language abilities within normal limits had undergone tumour resection only. The case reports of the four cases demonstrating language impairments are outlined briefly below.

Case 1 (Roger)

Roger was admitted to hospital at the age of 3;9 months. He was clumsy, had been irritable for 2 days and had experienced a mild weight loss. A neurological examination indicated bilateral papilloedema and inco-ordination to be the only abnormalities. A CT scan performed on admission revealed moderate hydrocephalus with dilation of the third and lateral ventricles associated with a mass lesion in the foramen magnum and fourth ventricle. A ventriculoperitoneal (VP) shunt was inserted and a posterior fossa craniotomy performed, resulting in the diagnosis of a medulloblastoma. A rapid recovery was reported and no immediate complications post-surgery were experienced. Mutism following surgery was not recorded. Roger underwent a course of radiotherapy to the whole brain and spinal cord. A CT scan performed 22 months post-surgery showed the presence of calcification in the temporal fossa, posterior temporal regions and frontal lobes (Figure 3.1) consistent with the effects of radiotherapy (see Chapter 2).

At the time of language assessment two years five months post-surgery, Roger presented as an alert, co-operative six-year-old child who was still attending pre-school as his teacher believed he was not ready for Grade 1. Roger achieved below average scores (i.e. standard score = 6,

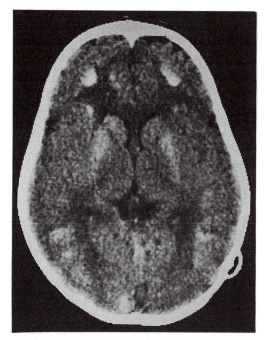

Figure 3.1 Roger: a CT scan performed 22 months post-surgery.

mean = 10, SD = 3) on the TOLD-P in the areas of expressive semantics (Oral Vocabulary Subtest), syntactic comprehension (Grammatical Understanding) and expressive syntax (Sentence Imitation). Scores for the areas of receptive vocabulary and auditory discrimination were within normal limits. Roger obtained a below average Overall Language Quotient and below average quotients for Speaking and Syntax. Other language quotients, however, were within normal limits.

Of the three CELF subtests administered, Producing Word Associations was performed above criterion in comparison to normative data provided in the test manual. Roger did not know the days of the week or the months of the year in order to complete the Producing Word Series task and was not familiar with the colours and shapes included in the Producing Names on Confrontation subtest. Therefore, he scored below criterion on these subtests. Overall, the language tests indicated that Roger had a mild language impairment with particular difficulties being experienced in the areas of expressive semantics and expressive and receptive syntax.

Several authors have linked the occurrence of intracerebral calcifications in children with the cranial irradiation and/or chemotherapy administered in cases of childhood cancer (Lee and Suh, 1977; Giralt et al., 1978; Hodges and Smithells, 1983; Pearson et al., 1983). Thus, it is possible that the language deficit exhibited by Roger represented a the

CELF (Subtests 7 and 8) further indicate the presence of an overall cognitive deficit. It is probable that the observed calcification is the product of the radiotherapy undergone by Roger when he was aged 3;9. Residual effects of the cortical compression associated with hydrocephalus may also be another factor contributing to the occurrence of the language disturbance.

It is difficult to assess whether the language problems observed in Roger reflect an acquired aphasia or an interruption to the normal developmental process of language acquisition, as the reduced syntactic ability, which has been observed in children with acquired aphasia (Alajouanine and Lhermitte, 1965; Satz and Bullard-Bates, 1981; Carrow-Woolfolk and Lynch, 1982; Van Dongen et al., 1985) is also frequently seen in cases of developmental language impairments (Aram and Nation, 1981).

Case 2 (Glen)

Glen was a boy aged 8;8. He had been admitted to hospital at the age of 2;7. On admission he was 'talking well' and developing normally but was listless, unco-ordinated and vomited daily. A neurological examination revealed bilateral papilloedema and dysfunction of the eighth cranial nerve. No other neurological abnormalities were recorded. A CT scan performed on admission showed a midline tumour in the posterior fossa arising from the cerebellum. It measured 3.5 cm in anterior–posterior diameter. Enlarged lateral and third ventricles due to obstructive hydrocephalus were also reported. An ependymoma was diagnosed. A VP shunt was inserted to alleviate the hydrocephalus and a posterior fossa craniotomy was performed. Glen had a left facial palsy following surgery which had not resolved at the time of his speech and language assessment at age 8;8. He was discharged from hospital 10 weeks after surgery following a course of radiotherapy which involved a total dose of 4000 rads to the whole brain and spinal cord. Glen spent a prolonged period (27 days) in the intensive care unit and was mute for 6 months following surgery. After this he made a particularly slow but uneventful recovery. A CT scan performed 3 years post-surgery demonstrated dramatic ventriculomegaly which was most marked in the fourth ventricle because of the fourth ventricle tumour resection (see Figure 3.2).

At the time of his language assessment, Glen was aged 8;8. He presented as a happy co-operative child who was enjoying Grade 1 at a small country school where he was receiving remedial instruction twice a week. Due to his ataxic gait, he required assistance when walking and wore a helmet to protect his head from frequent falls.

The results of the TOLD-P indicated the presence of a severe language delay with all subtests and quotients falling below the normal range. All three subtests of the CELF were scored below criterion. Glen did not know the days of the week or the months of the year in order to complete the Producing Word Series task and his dysarthria limited the speed at which he was able to complete the Producing Names on Confrontation and Producing Word Association subtests.

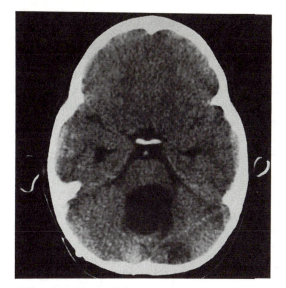

Figure 3.2 Glen: CT scan performed three years post-surgery.

Glen used telegraphic speech in the sentence imitation subtest of the TOLD-P, reproducing mainly content words. In spontaneous speech, utterances between five and eight words in length were unintelligible. Glen deliberately reduced such utterances to one or two words to enable the listener to comprehend his meaning. His receptive language skills (approximately six-year level) appeared to be in line with his academic functioning as a Grade 1 child as reported by his mother. Therefore, although Glen was impaired in all areas of language, the presence of a concomitant severe mixed dysarthria appeared also to contribute to his poor expressive language skills.

Overall, Glen evidenced a global language deficit involving all aspects of reception and expression. In the light of this child's delayed academic functioning, a full neuropsychological assessment would be required before the proper interpretation of these observed language results could be made, as cognitive deficits may also be present. Consideration of the tumour site does not lead to the prediction of a language disability, however, as has been mentioned, there are features secondary to the occurrence of a posterior fossa tumour that must be considered.

Although the presence of intracranial calcification was not evident in the CT scan performed three years post-surgery, calcification has been found to be a delayed reaction occurring between five and 14 years post-treatment (Giralt et al., 1978; Hodges and Smithells, 1983; Pearson et al., 1983; Lichtor et al., 1984). Cerebral radionecrosis is another late effect of cranial irradiation that has been documented. It refers to morphological changes in the brain tissue which are indicative of cell death and has been linked to the dose, time and fractionation of radio-therapy (Marks et al., 1981; Marks and Wong, 1985). In addition, cerebrovascular disease has been documented in children who have experienced radiotherapy (Painter et al., 1975; Wright and Bresnan, 1976).

Despite the lack of evidence of cortical abnormalities in his most recent CT scan, the presence of cerebral radionecrosis or radiation-induced cerebrovascular disease cannot be ruled out as possible contributors to the continuing speech and language disorders exhibited by Glen. Further, a considerable degree of hydrocephalus was noted at the time of admission, therefore, damage resulting from prolonged cortical compression may be another factor influencing his language functioning.

Case 3 (Ronald)

Ronald had a posterior fossa ependymoma removed when he was aged 2;1. The tumour measured 3.4 cm in diameter and was situated in the vermis passing towards the left side and downwards into the brainstem (Figure 3.3). A VP shunt was also inserted. Mutism was not reported to have occurred post-surgery. No post-surgical complications were experienced. Both radiotherapy and chemotherapy followed the surgical procedures. Three years post-surgery, Ronald received speech therapy for cluster reduction, final consonant deletion and progressive assimilation which were described as developmental in nature and not related to his surgical condition. There was no evidence of dysarthria at that time and both receptive and expressive skills were described as above average. Ronald's language abilities were assessed at age 8;10. He presented as a happy, energetic child who was small for his age.

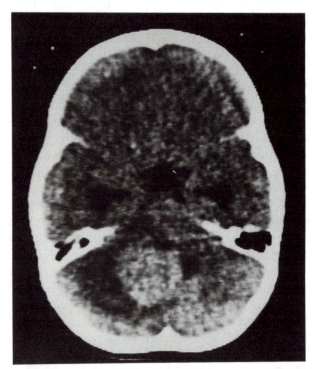

Figure 3.3 Ronald: CT scan showing location of a tumour situated in the vermis.

Scores achieved by Ronald on all subtests and quotients of the TOLD-P were within the normal range, suggesting that his overall language abilities were within normal limits. However, the Producing Word Associations subtest of the CELF was below criterion, suggesting the presence of a word retrieval problem since both picture and oral vocabulary scores were normal.

In summary, Ronald's overall language abilities were within normal limits, however, word retrieval problems were noted on his performance on the CELF. As discussed previously, delayed effects of irradiation and/or chemotherapy such as intracranial calcification, radionecrosis or cerebrovascular disease could be related to these observations, as could the residual effects of hydrocephalus. Further, the suggested word retrieval difficulties, in the absence of other language deficits, may have implications for Ronald's future educational success particularly as he attempts higher grades of schooling and, hence, his progress should be monitored. The large latency periods between the completion of radiotherapy and the onset of neurological symptoms recorded by several researchers (Lee and Suh, 1977; Giralt et al., 1978; Marks et al., 1981; Kearsley, 1983; Pearson et al., 1983), as well as the progressive nature of some delayed reactions, also have implications for the long-term monitoring required for individuals treated for posterior fossa tumours.

Case 4 (Edward)

Edward a male aged 15;4 was admitted to hospital at the age of 13 years. He had a history of headaches, a slight ataxia and a slight inco-ordination of the left hand. A CT scan performed on admission showed an infiltrating low density mass lesion in the cerebellum (Figure 3.4). It was in the midline, compressing the fourth ventricle from its dorsal aspect. Marked hydrocephalus with dilation of the third and lateral ventricles was also present. A VP shunt was inserted and one week later the tumour was partially removed. Diagnosis was that of an ependymoma. Immediately following surgery, truncal ataxia was observed but speech was described as clear. Recovery was rapid and Edward was discharged 6 days later. A course of radiotherapy followed in which a total dose of 5000 rads was delivered to the whole brain and spinal cord. A residual ependymoma in the superior vermian cistern and mild ventromegaly was evidenced on a CT scan taken 6 months post-surgery.

The results of the TOAL-2 showed that Edward had an average level of oral language mastery. The scores for Reading/Grammar, however, fell below the normal range. All three subtests of the CELF were above criterion. The results of a neuropsychological examination performed 13 months post-surgery indicated the presence of a mild impairment of memory for verbally presented material and for new learning in this modality. A mild to moderate impairment of memory for visually presented material and for learning in the visual modality was also noted

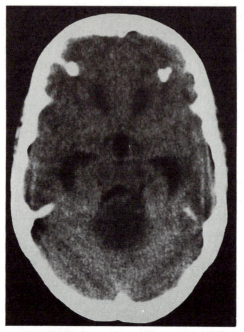

Figure 3.4 Edward: CT scan performed on admission showing an infiltrating low density mass lesion in the cerebellum.

along with a mild word finding difficulty. The Listening/Grammar subtest of the TOAL-2 requires the subject to listen to three sentences and choose the two which are closest in meaning. Edward demonstrated difficulty remembering the sentences he had heard. Difficulty was also experienced repeating the sentences in the Speaking/Grammar subtest.

Overall, despite the surgery, hydrocephalus and radiotherapy experienced, along with the presence of residual ependymoma and mild ventriculomegaly, Edward exhibited only a relatively mild language problem. In particular, his language abilities were shown to be adequate with the exception of reading ability. Reduced memory skills were also evident, reflecting a cognitive impairment possibly resulting from the effects of either radiotherapy or hydrocephalus.

In summary, the preliminary findings reported by Hudson et al. (1989) indicated that although language impairment is not the inevitable outcome of surgery to remove posterior fossa tumours in children, in some cases language deficits do occur. The linguistic deficits identified by Hudson et al. (1989), included deficits in the areas of expressive vocabulary and word finding, receptive syntax, expressive syntax and reading. Factors which could have influenced the language outcomes in the six cases reported included age at onset, tumour type, extent of surgical excision, the insertion of VP shunts, and the administration of radiotherapy and/or chemotherapy. In particular, Hudson et al. (1989) drew attention to the fact that the only two cases not to demonstrate language problems post-treatment, were those who had not received radiotherapy post-surgery.

Evidence from posterior fossa tumour group studies

As a follow-up to their earlier study, Hudson and Murdoch (1992) examined the language abilities of a group of children treated for brain tumours. Specifically, they compared the performance of a group of 20 paediatric tumour cases on a battery of language tests with that of a group of age- and sex-matched non-neurologically impaired control subjects. Their study represents the only group study of the chronic language abilities of children treated for posterior fossa tumours reported to date. The procedures utilized by Hudson and Murdoch (1992), with the major findings of their study, are outlined below.

The subjects examined by Hudson and Murdoch (1992), were 20 children who had been surgically treated for removal of a posterior fossa tumour at least 12 months previously. All subjects included were aged less than 15 years at the time of tumour diagnosis and treatment, and none had a pre-morbid history of birth trauma, head trauma, intellectual handicap, hearing loss, developmental delay, speech and/or language disorder, academic/learning deficits or other significant medical complaints. English was the primary language of all subjects included and none had experienced cerebral infarct or haemorrhage as a complication of the tumour or its treatment.

The personal and medical details of the 20 subjects involved in the study appear in Table 3.1. The subject group comprised 15 males and five females. A male:female ratio of 3:1 is representative of the general population in which up to three times as many boys than girls experience posterior fossa tumours (Russell and Rubinstein, 1989). All subjects were right-handed. At the time of tumour diagnosis, the subjects ranged in age from 1;9 to 13;3 ($M = 86.65 \pm 48.58$ months). Seven subjects were diagnosed with posterior fossa tumours when less than five years of age and, hence, had not yet attained all of the speech sounds and language structures of a mature communicator at the time of CNS trauma. Six subjects were aged between five and nine years at the time of tumour diagnosis, and the remaining seven were diagnosed when more than 10 years of age. Medical files indicated that all tumour cases included in the study reported by Hudson and Murdoch (1992) had evidence of occlusive hydrocephalus prior to surgery.

All 20 subjects underwent either biopsy (one subject) or partial (five subjects), subtotal (two subjects) or complete (12 subjects) tumour removal. Following surgery, four subjects (Cases 8, 13, 14 and 20) were reportedly mute for periods up to six months. A histological tumour diagnosis was confirmed in all 20 cases. Eight subjects had astrocytomas (three cystic, two juvenile, two solid and one unknown), five had ependymomas, six had medulloblastomas and one had a benign germinoma. Fourteen subjects received between 4000 and 5000 rads of radiotherapy, with one of those subjects also undergoing a course of chemotherapy. CNS prophylaxis was not included in the treatment protocols of five of the children diagnosed with astrocytoma as well as the child with the germinoma.

A comprehensive battery of standardized language assessments was selected in order to evaluate receptive and expressive semantic and syntactic skills as well as higher-level language proficiency. It was not possible for all subjects to complete all aspects of the test battery due to age constraints, sensory and/or motor disabilities, level of functional communicative ability, and/or the occurrence of medical complications or recurrent illness before completion of the study. Depending on their age at the time of testing, each subject was given one of the tests from the TOLD series, including the TOLD-P, TOLD-I or TOAL-2. The TOLD series was chosen as a general measure of a range of language skills which accommodates the large age range covered by the subjects while still allowing some comparisons to be made between subjects of different ages. Each test in the TOLD series provides an Overall Language Quotient as well as quotients for listening and speaking. The TOLD-P and TOLD-I also provide quotients for semantics and syntax, whereas the TOAL-2 considers eight language measures, including reading, writing, receptive and expressive vocabulary and grammar in spoken and written conditions, vocabulary, grammar, receptive language (spoken and written) and expressive language (spoken and written). In addition, to investigate rapid language retrieval and production each subject was also given the timed subtests of the CELF, including Subtest 7 — Producing Word Series, Subtest 8 — Producing Names on Confrontation and Subtest 9 – Producing Word Associations. The *Test of Language Competence* (TLC) (Wiig and Secord, 1985) was also included in the test battery utilized by Hudson and Murdoch (1992), to document advanced language competencies not assessed by standardized tests of semantics and syntax. The *Boston Naming Test* (BNT) (Kaplan, et al., 1983) was used to measure word-finding ability and, where appropriate, subjects were also given the *Token Test for Children* (DiSimoni, 1978) to further investigate auditory comprehension.

The results of the standardized language assessments administered by Hudson and Murdoch (1992) indicated that, as a group, children treated for posterior fossa tumour performed significantly below their peers on both receptive and expressive language tasks. The global measure of language ability provided by the Overall Language Quotients of the TOLD series indicated that, in the chronic stage post-treatment, children treated for posterior fossa tumour exhibit a level of language

Table 3.1 Biographical details of the 20 tumour subjects

Case	Sex	Age at assessment*	Age at diagnosis*	Time post-surgery*	Tumour type	Extent of surgery	Other treatments	Pre-surgical symptom duration**	Mute post-surgery?	Language status	Academic status
1	M	4;5	3;0	1;5	Epe	Total	R EVD	2	N	D	UA
2	F	5;10	3;2	2;8	Ast	Partial	R VPS	5	N	D	–
3	M	6;2	3;10	2;5	Med	Total	R VPS	2	N	D	+
4	F	6;3	5;1	1;2	Ast	Total	UA†	UA	N	WNL	–
5	M	7;1	5;9	1;5	Med	Total	R VPS	8	N	D	–
6	F	7;4	3;2	4;2	Ast	Subtotal	VPS†	3	N	D	–
7	M	7;5	1;9	5;8	Ast	Biopsy	R VPS	3	Y	D	–
8	M	8;8	2;7	6;1	Epe	Total	R VPS	12	N	D	+
9	M	9;6	7;2	2;4	Med	Partial	R VPS	2	N	WNL	–
10	M	11;1	7;4	3;9	Ast	Total	†	10	N	D	–
11	M	11;3	2;1	9;2	Epe	Partial	R C VPS	UA	N	D	+
12	M	11;4	9;9	1;8	Ger	Total	EVD†	2	N	D	–
13	M	13;4	11;3	2;1	Med	Total	R VPS	6	Y	D	–
14	F	12;10	10;6	2;5	Med	Total	R VPS	52	Y	D	–
15	M	13;1	10;10	2;3	Epe	Partial	R EVD	3	N	WNL	+
16	F	13;11	6;8	7;3	Ast	Total	VPS†	UA	N	WNL	+
17	M	14;11	13;0	1;11	Med	Subtotal	R	4	N	D	–
18	M	15;7	13;3	2;4	Epe	Partial	R VPS	8	N	D	+
19	M	16;1	12;3	3;10	Ast	Total	R	4	N	WNL	–
20	M	16;10	12;0	4;9	Ast	Total	VPS†	24	Y	D	–

*Years;months.

**Weeks.

† No CNS prophylaxis required.

M = Male; F = female.

Ast = Astrocytoma; Epe = ependymoma; Ger = germinoma; Med = medulloblastoma; C = chemotherapy; R = radiotherapy; EVD = external ventricular drain; VPS = ventriculoperitoneal shunt; UA = unavailable information; D = some language difficulty evident; N = no; WNL = within normal limits; Y = yes; + = performing adequately in a normal classroom situation; – = requiring academic assistance.

competence which is below that of a matched control group. Hudson and Murdoch (1992) noted, however, that the mean Overall Language Quotient of 89 obtained by their tumour subjects was within the normal range of 85–115 specified in the tests' manuals. Thus, as a group, the children treated for tumour evidenced a mild language disturbance which the authors could describe as 'subclinical' in nature. Subclinical language difficulties were also documented by Jordan et al. (1988) who used the TOLD series to evaluate the long-term linguistic abilities of 20 children who had suffered either a mild or severe CHI. Although the CHI subjects achieved a mean Overall Language Quotient which was within the normal range of the tests, they performed significantly below a matched control group. Jordan et al. (1988) suggested that the CHI subjects in their study exhibited a 'subclinical aphasia'.

Unfortunately, neuropsychological measures were not recorded by Hudson and Murdoch (1992) and consequently these authors were unable to determine whether the language disturbances observed in their tumour group were purely aphasic in nature or whether cognitive and language deficits were co-occurring. Examination of individual tumour cases, however, demonstrated that half the tumour subjects (Cases 1, 2, 3, 5, 10, 11, 12, 13, 18 and 20) exhibited specific language disabilities rather than a global reduction across all language skills.

As a group, the children treated for posterior fossa tumour also exhibited reduced auditory comprehension abilities relative to the control group. Studies reported to date have implicated radiotherapy as the factor responsible for the auditory recall and auditory comprehension deficits experienced by children who have undergone treatments for posterior fossa tumour (Painter et al., 1975; Lansky et al., 1984; Taylor et al., 1987; Packer et al., 1989). Despite the finding by Hudson and Murdoch (1992) of reduced comprehension abilities in the tumour group, the administration of CNS irradiation was not shown by these authors to be a primary causal factor. The 14 tumour subjects in their study who had experienced CNS irradiation were found to not differ significantly from the five tumour subjects who underwent surgery only when compared on the Listening Quotient of the TOLD series. This finding suggests that other factors common to all posterior fossa tumour patients, such as hydrocephalus, an interruption to development, or emotional effects may also be factors that influence the long-term comprehension skills of this population.

Hudson and Murdoch (1992) also failed to identify a difference in the receptive abilities of those children aged less than five years when the tumour was diagnosed. Several authors have determined age at the time of neurological incident to be an important prognostic indicator for comprehension skills (Alajouanine and Lhermitte, 1965; Vargha-Khadem et al., 1985; Aram and Ekelman, 1987). A study by Lansky et al. (1984) determined that for leukaemia/lymphoma patients who received CNS chemotherapy and radiotherapy, the younger the age at diagnosis, the lower the verbal intelligence quotient (VIQ) and comprehension scores. This finding is consistent with reports that children aged less than five years at the time of CNS irradiation are more likely to exhibit structural damage to the CNS in the long term (Pearson et al., 1983; Davis et al., 1986).

A mild reduction in expressive language abilities was also characteristic of the posterior fossa tumour group investigated by Hudson and Murdoch (1992). The syntactic abilities (both expressive and receptive) of the subjects who completed either the TOLD-P or TOLD-I were also noted by these authors to be mildly impaired. A reduction in the quantity and complexity of language output has been widely reported in children suffering a range of acquired neurological disorders and has often been associated with a period of mutism immediately post-injury (Alajouanine and Lhermitte, 1965; Hécaen, 1983; Van Dongen et al., 1985; Aram et al., 1986; Cooper and Flowers, 1987; Jordan et al., 1988; Basso and Scarpa, 1990). Only four of the 20 tumour subjects examined by Hudson and Murdoch (1992) exhibited mutism immediately post-surgery. A psychological or emotional basis for the occurrence of mutism post-injury has been proposed (Byers and McLean, 1962; Alajouanine and Lhermitte, 1965), however, mutism following CNS trauma has also been reported to precede the onset of dysarthria (Hécaen, 1983; Rekate et al., 1985; Volcan et al., 1986) as occurred in each of the four cases who were mute post-surgery and examined by Hudson and Murdoch (1992). Their findings indicated that a lack of mutism post-surgery does not necessarily imply intact language skills in the long term.

Perhaps the most frequently reported language deficits associated with acquired neurological aetiologies relate to naming skills. Hudson and Murdoch (1992) failed to detect deficient confrontation naming abilities in their group of tumour cases as determined by the BNT and the CELF (Subtest 8). Reduced naming scores as well as the presence of semantic, phonemic and neologistic paraphasic errors are characteristic of acquired language disorders, even in the absence of other language deficits (Carter et al., 1982; Van Dongen et al., 1985; Van Hout et al., 1985; Cooper and Flowers, 1987; Jordan et al., 1988; Lees and Neville, 1990). Painter et al. (1975) identified anomia in a nine-year-old girl two years after undergoing surgery and irradiation for a cerebellar medulloblastoma. Symptoms were associated with a mass in the left posterior temporal lobe, a late-delayed reaction of CNS irradiation.

The rapid retrieval and production of language abilities was not reported to be significantly impaired in the group of children treated for posterior fossa tumours examined by Hudson and Murdoch (1992). However, these authors did note a range of retrieval and production abilities within the tumour group. This finding contrasts with that of several neuropsychological studies in which children who had received CNS radiotherapy for the treatment of brain tumours or acute lymphoblastic leukaemia exhibited deficits in word fluency and rapid contingency naming (Brouwers et al., 1985; Taylor et al., 1987; Packer et al., 1989).

The reading and writing abilities of the six tumour cases who completed the TOAL-2 were reported by Hudson and Murdoch (1992) to be within normal limits and not significantly different from the control group. Moderate to severe reading, writing and spelling difficulties have been identified in children who experienced a wide range of lesion types and sites (Alajouanine and Lhermitte, 1965; Hécaen, 1976; Carter et al., 1982; Van Dongen et al., 1985; Cooper and Flowers, 1987; Basso and Scarpa, 1990; Lees and Neville, 1990). In particular, Hécaen (1976) determined that children who experienced a rapid onset lesion (e.g. traumatic brain injury) were prone to writing disturbances. The CNS trauma experienced by the subjects in the study reported by Hudson and Murdoch (1992) occurred over an extended period of time which may account for their intact writing abilities. Age at onset may also have influenced writing ability. Alajouanine and Lhermitte (1965) determined severe writing disturbances in all nine of their subjects who experienced a left cerebral lesion when less than 10 years of age. Five of the six children treated for brain tumours reported by Hudson and Murdoch (1992) were older than 10 years when diagnosed and treated for their condition. It is possible that the reading and writing skills acquired prior to the diagnosis and treatment of a posterior fossa tumour are retained and extended in the long term.

The mild language disturbances detected by the test battery employed by Hudson and Murdoch (1992) indicate that, as a group, children treated for posterior fossa tumour may not be competent language users when compared to their peers. The TLC results reported by Hudson and Murdoch (1992) confirmed previous test results, indicating deficiencies in the understanding and manipulation of complex and abstract language structures. The investigation of high-level language skills in children with acquired neurological disorders is limited. Cooper and Flowers (1987) concluded that their 15 subjects of mixed aetiologies exhibited deficits that 'most characteristically occurred in later developing syntactic and metalinguistic abilities' (p. 261). Complete resolution of acquired language deficits is no longer considered to be an inevitable outcome of acquired brain lesions in childhood. With increasing reports of long-term word-finding difficulties, reading, writing and spelling deficits, and reduced receptive and expressive language skills (e.g. Hécaen, 1976; Van Dongen et al., 1985; Jordan et al., 1988; Lees and Neville, 1990), the risk of high-level language deficits and their effects on academic performance in children with acquired brain lesions need further investigation.

Although the administration of CNS prophylaxis has been reported to affect the long-term functional abilities of paediatric cancer patients

(Meadows et al., 1981; Danoff et al., 1982; Silverman et al., 1984; Copeland et al., 1985; Duffner et al., 1985), the 14 irradiated subjects investigated by Hudson and Murdoch (1992) did not perform differently from the six children in their study who did not receive CNS irradiation on overall, listening and speaking language tasks. In the descriptive study of six children who had been treated for posterior fossa tumour reported by Hudson et al. (1989), language difficulties were identified in the four children who had received CNS irradiation, whereas the two children who only experienced surgery exhibited intact language abilities. The findings reported by Hudson and Murdoch (1992), however, were less conclusive. Four of the six subjects in the latter study with intact language had received CNS irradiation and four of the six subjects who did not require CNS prophylaxis demonstrated at least some degree of language difficulty. Thus, although radiotherapy may influence post-treatment language abilities, other factors must also influence language performance in the long term.

Tumour type also did not appear to influence the performance of children treated for posterior fossa tumours on language tasks in the study reported by Hudson and Murdoch (1992). In that the administration of CNS prophylaxis is usually dependent upon the type of tumour that is diagnosed, it could be expected that astrocytoma subjects would demonstrate superior language skills when compared to medulloblastoma and ependymoma subjects, both of whom require treatment with CNS prophylaxis (see Chapter 1). For example, Riva et al. (1989) determined reduced Full Scale IQs and VIQs in eight medulloblastoma patients when compared to seven astrocytoma patients and a sibling control group. The performance differences were attributed to the administration of radiotherapy in the treatment of medulloblastoma. In the Hudson and Murdoch (1992) study, three of the eight subjects treated for astrocytoma required craniospinal irradiation. This may have negatively influenced the language scores of their astrocytoma group.

All of the tumour cases examined by Hudson and Murdoch (1992) had symptoms of occlusive hydrocephalus before surgery. In that the pre-operative duration of hydrocephalus (i.e. the duration of symptoms such as headache, vomiting, diplopia etc.) may be an important factor influencing cognitive outcome following posterior fossa pathology, these authors correlated the duration of pre-surgical hydrocephalus with the Overall, Listening and Speaking Language Quotients recorded for each tumour subject. A significant correlation, however, was not determined. In a study of a group of 38 brain tumour patients, Danoff et al. (1982) failed to relate the presence or absence of hydrocephalus to the occurrence of mental retardation.

The time that has elapsed since tumour onset is a variable that may influence language outcome. This variable, however, was not examined by Hudson and Murdoch (1992). Their subjects were assessed from 14 months to seven years three months post-surgery. Evidence is available to suggest that the negative consequences of posterior fossa tumours and, in particular, CNS prophylaxis may develop up to 14 years after the completion of treatment (Painter et al., 1975; Lee and Suh, 1977; Burns and Boyle, 1984). This is an issue which has serious implications for the long-term well-being of tumour patients. Consequently, long-term changes in language and neuropsychological performances over time require extensive investigation utilizing a large subject group in order to determine prognostic implications for this population.

Management of language disorders subsequent to paediatric brain tumours

The findings of case studies as well as group studies reported in the literature to date indicate that, although not inevitable, language disorders do occur in children in the chronic stage subsequent to treatment for posterior fossa tumours. Further, it is clear that all aspects of language may be compromised in this population and hence, there is a need to monitor both the receptive and expressive language abilities of children treated for posterior fossa tumours throughout their school years.

As yet, no characteristic language pattern has been elucidated to provide clinicians with a starting point for patient management, or to alert them to specific areas of language deficit that may require more in-depth evaluation in tumour cases. Rather, the data available to date indicate the presence of variable language abilities within the tumour population thereby necessitating the need for development and implementation of individualized therapy programmes. Although sharing a common aetiology (i.e. posterior fossa tumour), because they represent a variety of tumour types requiring different treatment approaches, children treated for posterior fossa tumours do not represent a homogeneous group. For instance, it is apparent that several complicating factors, such as CNS irradiation, chemotherapy, hydrocephalus etc., may also influence the long-term language abilities of posterior fossa tumour patients, although as yet the precise contribution of these factors to the manifestation of language disorders is unknown. Consequently, therapy for this population can never be prescriptive as it is essential that clinicians evaluate each child's abilities in the context of the tumour treatment being given (e.g., surgery, radiotherapy, chemotherapy), the presence of other complicating factors (such as hydrocephalus and VP shunts), the presence of any intellectual deterioration, the educational status of the child, the involvement of other medical and educational services and the emotional state of the child and their family.

It is noteworthy that neurological deterioration can occur from months to years after the completion of treatment of brain tumours

(Kun et al., 1983; Silverman et al., 1984; Mulhern and Kun, 1985) (see Chapter 2). Consequently, clinicians need to be aware of the need to obtain initial baseline measurements of language abilities from these children and to review them at six- or 12-monthly intervals for several years whether or not speech pathology was recommended subsequent to the initial assessment. Speech and language pathologists, therefore, need to take an active role in the management of children treated for brain tumours, even if initially intervention does not appear warranted. In particular, the high-level language skills that may influence academic performance should be monitored and, if necessary, the appropriate intervention provided.

References

Alajouanine T, Lhermitte F (1965) Acquired aphasia in children. Brain 88: 653–662.

Aram D, Nation J (1981) Child Language Disorders. New York: Mosby.

Aram DM, Ekelman BL (1987) Unilateral brain lesions in childhood: performance on the Revised Token Test. Brain and Language 323: 127–158.

Aram DM, Ekelman BL, Whitaker HA (1986) Spoken syntax in children with acquired unilateral hemisphere lesions. Brain and Language 27: 75–100.

Bamford FN, Morris-Jones P, Pearson D, Ribeiro GG, Shalet SM, Beardwell CG (1976) Residual disabilities in children treated for intracranial space-occupying lesions. Cancer 37: 1149–1151.

Basso A, Scarpa T (1990) Traumatic aphasia in children and adults: a comparison of clinical features and evolution. Cortex 26: 501–514.

Broadbent VA, Barnes ND, Wheeler TK (1981) Medulloblastoma in childhood: long-term results of treatment. Cancer 48: 26–30.

Brouwers P, Riccardi R, Fedio P, Poplack DG (1985) Long-term neuropsychologic sequelae of childhood leukemia: correlation with CT brain scan abnormalities. Journal of Pediatrics 106: 723–728.

Burns MS, Boyle M (1984) Aphasia after successful radiation treatment: a report of two cases (Letter to the Editor). Journal of Speech and Hearing Disorders 49: 107–111.

Byers RK, McLean WT (1962) Etiology and course of certain hemiplegias with aphasia in childhood. Pediatrics 29: 376–38.

Carrow-Woolfolk E, Lynch J (1982) An Integrated Approach to Language Disorders in Children. Orlando, FL: Grune & Stratton.

Carter RL, Hohenegger MK, Satz P (1982) Aphasia and speech organization in children. Science 218: 797–799.

Cooper JA, Flowers CR (1987) Children with a history of acquired aphasia: residual language and academic impairments. Journal of Speech and Hearing Disorders 52: 251–262.

Copeland DR, Fletcher JM, Pfefferbaum-Levine B, Jaffe N, Reid H, Maor M (1985) Neuropsychological sequelae of childhood cancer in long-term survivors. Pediatrics 75: 745–753.

Danoff BF, Chowchock FS, Marquette C, Mulgrew L, Kramer S (1982) Assessment of the long-term effects of primary radiation therapy for brain tumours in children. Cancer 49: 1580–1586.

Davis PC, Hoffman JC, Pearl GS, Braun IF (1986) CT evaluation of effects of cranial radiation therapy in children. American Journal of Roentgenology 147: 587–592.

DiSimoni F (1978) The Token Test for Children. Hingham, MA: Teaching Resources.

Duffner PK, Cohen ME, Thomas PRM (1983) Late effects of treatment on the intelligence of children with posterior fossa tumours. Cancer 51: 233–237.

Duffner PK, Cohen ME, Thomas RM, Lansky SB (1985) The long-term effects of cranial irradiation on the central nervous system. Cancer 56: 1841–1846.

Giralt M, Gil JL, Borderas F, Oliveros A, Gomez-Pereda R, Pardo J, Martinez-Ibanez F, Raichs A (1978) Intracerebral calcifications in childhood lymphoblastic leukemia. Acta Haematologica 59: 193–204.

Hammill DD, Newcomer PL (1982). Test of Language Development — Intermediate. Austin, TX: Pro-Ed.

Hammill DD, Brown VL, Larsen SC, Wiederhold JL (1987) Test of Adolescent Language 2: A Multidimensional Approach to Assessment. Austin, TX: Pro-Ed.

Hécaen H (1976) Acquired aphasia in children and the otogenesis of hemispheric functional specialization. Brain and Language 3: 114–134.

Hécaen H (1983) Acquired aphasia in children: revisited. Neuropsychologia 21: 581–587.

Hodges S, Smithells RW (1983) Intercranial calcification and childhood medulloblastoma. Archives of Disease in Childhood 58: 663–664.

Hudson LJ, Murdoch BE (1992) Chronic language deficits in children treated for posterior fossa tumours. Aphasiology 6: 135–150.

Hudson LJ, Murdoch BE, Ozanne AE (1989) Posterior fossa tumours in childhood: associated speech and language disorders post-surgery. Aphasiology 3: 1–18.

Jordan FM, Ozanne AE, Murdoch BE (1988) Long term speech and language disorders subsequent to closed head injury in children. Brain Injury 2: 179–185.

Kadota RP, Allen JB, Hartman GA, Spruce WE (1989) Brain tumors in children. Journal of Pediatrics 114: 511–519.

Kaplan E, Goodglass H, Weintraub S (1983) Boston Naming Test. Philadelphia, PA: Lea & Febiger.

Kearsley JH (1983) Late cerebrovascular disease after radiation therapy: report of two cases and a review of the literature. Australasian Radiology 27: 11–18.

Kun LE, Mulhern RK, Crisco JJ (1983) Quality of life in children treated for brain tumour. Journal of Neurosurgery 58: 1–6.

Lansky SB, Cairns NU, Lansky LL, Cairns GF, Stephenson L, Garin G (1984) Central nervous system prophylaxis: studies showing impairment in verbal skills and academic achievement. American Journal of Pediatric Hematology/Oncology 6: 183–190.

Lee KF, Suh JH (1977) CT evidence of grey matter calcification secondary to radiation therapy. Computerized Tomography 1: 103–110.

Lees JA, Neville BGR (1990) Acquired aphasia in childhood: case studies of five children. Aphasiology 4: 463–478.

Lichtor T, Wollmann RL, Brown FD (1984) Calcified basal ganglionic mass 12 years after radiation therapy for medulloblastoma. Surgical Neurology 21: 373–376.

Marks JE, Wong J (1985) The risk of cerebral radionecrosis in relation to dose, time and fractionation. Progress in Experimental Tumour Research 29: 210–218.

Marks JE, Baglan RJ, Prassad SC, Blank WF (1981) Cerebral radionecrosis: incidence and risk in relation to dose, time, fractionation and volume. International Journal of Radiation Oncology, Biology and Physics 7: 243–252.

Meadows AT, Massari DJ, Ferguson J, Gordon J, Littman P, Moss K (1981) Declines in IQ scores and cognitive dysfunctions in children with acute lymphocytic leukaemia treated with cranial irradiation. Lancet ii: 1015–1018.

Miller JF, Campbell TF, Chapman RS, Weismer SE (1984) Language behaviour in acquired childhood aphasia. In Holland A (ed.) Language Disorders in Children. Baltimore, MD: College-Hill Press: 55–99.

Mulhern RK, Kun LE (1985) Neuropsychologic function in children with brain tumours. III. Interval changes in the six months following treatment. Medical and Pediatric Oncology 13: 318–324.

Murdoch BE, Hudson-Tennent LJ (1994) Differential language outcomes in children following treatment for posterior fossa tumours. Aphasiology 8: 507–534.

Newcomer PL, Hammill DD (1982). Test of Language Development — Primary. Austin, TX: Pro-Ed.

Packer RJ, Sutton LN, Atkins TE, Radcliffe J, Bunin GR, D'Angio G, Seigel KR, Schut L (1989) A prospective study of cognitive function in children receiving whole-brain radiotherapy and chemotherapy: 2-year results. Journal of Neurosurgery 70: 707–713.

Painter MJ, Chutorian AM, Hilal SK (1975) Cerebrovasculopathy following irradiation in childhood. Neurology 25: 189–194.

Pearson ADJ, Campbell AN, McAllister VL, Pearson GL (1983) Intracranial calcification in survivors of childhood medulloblastoma. Archives of Disease in Childhood 58: 133–136.

Rekate HL, Grubb RL, Aram DM, Hahn JF, Ratcheson RA (1985) Muteness of cerebellar origin. Archives of Neurology 42: 697–698.

Riva D, Pantaleoni C, Milani N, Fossati Belani F (1989) Impairment of neuropsychological functions in children with medulloblastomas and astrocytomas in the posterior fossa. Child's Nervous System 5: 107–110.

Russell DS, Rubinstein LJ (1989) Pathology of Tumours of the Nervous System (fifth edition). London: Edward Arnold.

Satz P, Bullard-Bates C (1981) Acquired aphasia in children. In Sarno MT (ed.) Acquired Aphasia. New York: Academic Press: 398–426.

Segall HD, Batnitzky S, Zee S, Ahmadi J, Bird CR, Cohen ME (1985) Computed tomography in the diagnosis of intracranial neoplasms in children. Cancer 56: 1748–1755.

Semel EM, Wiig EH (1982) Clinical Evaluation of Language Functions. Columbus, OH: Charles E Merrill.

Silverman CL, Palkes H, Talent B, Kovnar E, Clouse JW, Thomas PRM (1984) Late effects of radiotherapy on patients with cerebellar medulloblastoma. Cancer 54: 825–829.

Taylor HG, Albo VC, Phebus CK, Sachs BR, Bierl PG (1987) Postirradiation treatment outcomes for children with acute lymphocytic leukaemia: clarification of risks. Journal of Pediatric Psychology 12: 395–411.

Van Dongen HR, Loonen CB, Van Dongen KJ (1985) Anatomical basis for acquired fluent aphasia in children. Annals of Neurology 17: 306–309.

Van Hout A, Evrard P, Lyon G (1985) On the positive semiology of acquired aphasia in children. Developmental Medicine and Child Neurology 27: 231–241.

Vargha-Khadem F, Gorman AM, Watters GV (1985) Aphasia and handedness in relation to hemispheric side, age and injury and severity of cerebral lesion during childhood. Brain 108: 677–696.

Volcan I, Cole GP, Johnston K (1986) A case of muteness of cerebellar origin. Archives of Neurology 43: 313–314.

Wiig EH, Secord W (1985) Test of Language Competence. Columbus, OH: Charles E Merrill.

Wright TL, Bresnan MJ (1976) Radiation induced cerebrovascular disease in children. Neurology 26: 540–543.

Chapter 4
Language recovery following treatment for paediatric brain tumours

BRUCE E MURDOCH AND LISA J HUDSON

Introduction

In earlier chapters of this book (see Chapters 2 and 3) it has been established that paediatric cancer patients, including children treated for posterior fossa tumours, are at risk of developing structural and functional deficits in the central nervous system (CNS). Structural changes to the nervous system as a result of CNS radiotherapy and/or chemotherapy include necrosis, calcification and demyelination and have been detected in both the white and grey matter of the cerebral and cerebellar hemispheres (Lee and Suh, 1977; Marks et al., 1981; Pearson et al., 1983; Lichtor et al., 1984; Davis et al., 1986; Dooms et al., 1986; Price et al., 1988). In addition, generalized cerebral and cerebellar atrophy and cerebrovascular disease may also develop after the completion of CNS prophylaxis (De Reuck and vander Eecken, 1975; Painter et al., 1975; Wright and Bresnan, 1976; Lichtor et al., 1984; Curnes et al., 1986; Davis et al., 1986; Price et al., 1988) (see Chapter 2).

Functional changes in the CNS reported to occur as long-term complications of the surgery, radiotherapy and chemotherapy experienced by children treated for brain tumours include various neurological, neuropsychological, speech and language deficits. Particular disabilities that have been documented include dysarthria, receptive and expressive language deficits in the areas of syntax and semantics, intellectual deficits, memory deficits, learning disabilities, ataxia, hemiplegia, cranial nerve palsies and visual and hearing impairments (Painter et al., 1975; Broadbent et al., 1981; Marks et al., 1981; Danoff et al., 1982; Silverman et al., 1984; Brouwers et al., 1985; Duffner et al., 1985; Hudson et al., 1989; Hudson and Murdoch, 1992a, b; Murdoch and Hudson-Tennent, 1994).

In general, improvement in the language abilities of children with acquired aphasia is considered to be more rapid and complete than in adults. Alajouanine and Lhermitte (1965) reported recovery in two-thirds of their children when reassessed at least 12 months after injury. Although Carrow-Woolfolk and Lynch (1982) observed that children under 10 years of age have a fair chance of reacquiring verbal skills within one year, Alajouanine and Lhermitte (1965) did not find a significant difference in the speed of recovery between children less than 10 years of age and children aged 10 or more years. The recovery of aphasia has been related to the cause, the site, the extent and the reversibility of the cerebral lesion (Alajouanine and Lhermitte, 1965; Van Dongen and Loonen, 1977) as well as to the age at injury (Satz and Bullard-Bates, 1981). Although, based on the above general assumption it could be expected that children with language disabilities associated with treatment for brain tumours would show considerable improvement over time, there are several factors related to the treatment process they experience that might make their prognosis for recovery different to that of children with acquired language disorders of different aetiology. For instance, evidence is available to suggest that structural and functional damage to the CNS following radiotherapy and/or chemotherapy does not always resolve spontaneously but is long term and perhaps very importantly even progressive in nature. For example, Price et al. (1988) examined the computerized tomographic (CT) scans of a nine-year-old child 23 months and 32 months post-irradiation and found evidence to suggest that calcification of the brain occurring subsequent to irradiation is progressive in nature. Tsuruda et al. (1987) also implicated progressive deterioration in cases of radiation-related CNS damage. After comparing the magnetic resonance imaging (MRI) scans of 95 patients who had been irradiated for a wide variety of CNS tumours with the MRI scans of 180 age-matched control subjects, Tsuruda et al. (1987) concluded that the white matter changes that followed CNS irradiation represented the normal aging process but at an accelerated rate.

Although it has been reported that younger children with acquired aphasia have a more favourable prognosis than older children (Carrow-Woolfolk and Lynch, 1982), it is possible that the reverse is true in children who experience surgery and CNS prophylaxis for the treatment of brain tumours. Although detailed prospective studies documenting the pattern of language recovery of children treated for brain tumours are yet to be reported, studies of intellectual functioning have suggested that children with tumours who are less than six years of age at diagnosis and treatment have a greater risk of intellectual deterioration than those older than six years (Danoff et al., 1982; Mulhern and Kun, 1985). Whether or not a deterioration in language abilities parallels the reported decline in intellectual functioning has yet to be determined.

To gain some insight into the possible language recovery patterns demonstrated by children treated for brain tumours, the present chapter outlines the language changes documented by Hudson and Murdoch (1992a) in three children who experienced surgery and CNS irradiation for the treatment of posterior fossa medulloblastoma.

Case reports

The three cases reported below were selected on the basis that they exhibited a uniform tumour type (i.e. medulloblastoma). In addition, each child had also undergone the surgical insertion of a ventriculoperitoneal (VP) shunt to drain excess fluid from the lateral ventricles, and a six-week course of radiotherapy post-surgery. Throughout the duration of language monitoring, none of the three cases exhibited evidence of residual or recurrent tumour as demonstrated by regular (six-monthly) CT scans. The sex, age at diagnosis, radiation dose, number of language assessments and other relevant characteristics pertaining to each subject are outlined in Table 4.1.

Table 4.1 Characteristics of the three subjects treated for medulloblastoma

Subjects	1	2	3
Sex	F	M	M
Age at diagnosis*	10;6	7;2	5;9
Extent of surgical removal	Subtotal	Subtotal	Total
Radiation dose (rads)	5000	5000	4800
No. of language assessments	4	4	3
Presence/absence of dysarthria	Ataxic/flaccid	Absent	Absent
Pre-morbid school attainment	Grade 5	Grade 2	Grade 1
Handedness	R	R	R

*Age (years;months) (from Hudson and Murdoch, 1992a).

All three subjects had been attending normal primary schools prior to diagnosis, and according to pre-morbid school reports, had been performing at average or above average levels in all areas. All three subjects were right-handed. The subjects had no history of birth trauma, head trauma, intellectual handicap, learning disability, speech, language, and/or hearing deficits or other neurological disorders prior to diagnosis.

The language abilities of each subject were initially evaluated towards the end of the course of radiotherapy. Studies examining the long-term effects of tumour treatment on neuropsychological abilities have used the initial post-treatment assessment as the baseline for evaluating future changes in performance as objective information on pre-treatment abilities is rarely available (e.g. Kun et al., 1983; Packer et al., 1989). The subjects were then re-assessed at approximately six-monthly intervals thereafter.

The test battery used to monitor the language abilities of each subject included:

- Either the *Test of Language Development — Primary* (TOLD-P) (Newcomer and Hammill, 1982) or the *Test of Language Development – Intermediate* (TOLD-I) (Hammill and Newcomer, 1982) depending on the child's age at the time of testing. The TOLD series of tests was chosen to accommodate each subject's increasing age throughout the duration of the study. Subjects can move on to the next test in the series at the appropriate age while still allowing direct comparisons to be made with their earlier language performances. In addition, the recovery pattern over time of children of different ages can be compared.
- The *Boston Naming Test* (BNT) (Kaplan et al., 1983) was administered at each assessment to evaluate the subjects' semantic–lexical abilities. The presence of word-finding difficulties and paraphasias can be identified using this test.
- The *Token Test for Children* (DiSimoni, 1978) was administered at each child's final assessment to further examine language comprehension abilities.

Case 1 (Jane)

Case 1, (Jane) aged 10;6, underwent the surgical insertion of a VP shunt and extensive but subtotal excision of a posterior fossa medulloblastoma. This procedure resulted in a left divergent strabismis, a left hemiparesis and a left lower motor neurone facial palsy involving cranial nerve VII.

Post-operatively, Jane was able to speak up until the fifth day. She was then mute for 5 days, after which the only vocalizations she made included 'yeah', screaming, and a 'sad, sorrowing' sound. These inappropriate vocalizations continued for a further 10 days. Jane was then echolalic for approximately 2 weeks. A mixed ataxic/flaccid dysarthria was diagnosed 6 weeks post-surgery. This resolved spontaneously to a mild, primarily flaccid dysarthria and did not affect her intelligibility during the assessment period.

Jane's performance on the TOLD-I is detailed in Table 4.2. The first administration of the TOLD-I produced neither an overall Spoken Language Quotient, nor Speaking and Syntax Quotients because Jane was unable to understand the instructions or follow the examples given for the Word Ordering Subtest (see Table 4.2). Consequently, this task was omitted, leaving only two language quotients that could be calculated. The quotients obtained included a Listening Quotient of 76, which is below average, and a Semantics Quotient of 64, which is classified as a 'poor' language score according to the test's normative data (see Table 4.2). During administration of the TOLD-I, the presence of marked word-finding difficulties was observed.

Table 4.2 Case 1 (Jane): Language quotients and subtest standard scores obtained on the *Test of Language Development — Intermediate* (TOLD-I)

Test	Time post-surgery	SLQ	LiQ	SpQ	SeQ	SyQ	SC	Ch	WO	Gen	GC
1	6 weeks	NA	76*	NA	64**	NA	7	3*	NA	5*	9
2	7.5 months	75*	82*	74*	85	72*	4*	6*	5*	9	8
3	16 months	77*	79*	79*	79*	79*	9	6*	4*	7	7
4	20 months	79*	82*	81*	79*	83*	8	6*	6*	7	8

Note: Quotients: mean = 100, SD = 15; subtest standard scores: mean = 10, SD = 3
SLQ = Spoken Language Quotient; LiQ = Listening Quotient; SpQ = Speaking Quotient; SeQ = Semantics Quotient; SyQ = Syntax Quotient; SC = Sentence Combining Subtest; Ch = Characteristics Subtest; WO = Word Ordering Subtest; Gen = Generals Subtest; GC = Grammatic Comprehension Subtest.
NA = Not available.
* Below average result. ** Poor result (from Hudson and Murdoch, 1992a).

At the time of the second assessment one and a half months later Jane was temporarily residing in a home for handicapped children where she was receiving speech therapy, occupational therapy, physiotherapy and special education services. She demonstrated an increased level of alertness and interaction than was observed at the initial assessment. Improvements were recorded for the Listening and Semantics Quotients, however, the overall Spoken Language Quotient, and the Listening, Speaking and Syntax Quotients were still below the average range of 85–115 (see Table 4.2).

As the family was lost to follow-up for several months, the third speech and language evaluation was performed eight and a half months after the second. At this time, Jane presented as an outgoing, highly cooperative child who was repeating Grade 6. Difficulties with all school subjects were reported. She still exhibited a residual left facial paresis, a left hemiparesis, limb ataxia and divergent strabismus.

Administration of the TOLD-I revealed that Jane's listening, speaking, semantic and syntactic abilities were all at an equivalent level of competency, with a quotient of 79 being obtained for each aspect of language functioning (see Table 4.2). This suggests that Jane's language performance stabilized as the time that elapsed since tumour treatment increased. Marked improvements in performance, however, were not a feature of the recovery process. At the time of the third assessment, word-finding difficulties associated with frequent circumlocutory behaviour had not resolved since the initial TOLD-I administration.

All of the scores obtained at the fourth assessment (20 months) indicated that Jane still had a level of language competency which was below the average range expected from a 12-year-old child. A sample of Jane's written work also reflected impaired language abilities, with spelling and grammatical errors being prolific throughout the short sample. Pre-morbid school reports, and reports by Jane's mother, did not suggest the presence of any pre-treatment difficulties with language or with any other school subjects.

Thus, four administrations of the TOLD-I over a 19-month period demonstrated that Jane maintained relatively static levels of language performance over this period. Minimal improvements and performance stabilization were noted, however, Jane's language abilities remained below average.

Administration of the BNT at each of the four assessment sessions revealed below average scores of 31, 35 and 36 out of a possible 60 responses at the first three speech and language evaluations, and an average score of 38 at the fourth administration. The progressive improvement recorded in the BNT scores reflects resolution of the marked word finding difficulties observed initially (although difficulties were still observed during the final testing session), and confirms the improvement noted in the Semantics Quotient of the TOLD-I (see Table 4.2) over the same time period.

The *Token Test for Children*, administered at the fourth assessment only, indicated slightly below average receptive language abilities with an overall scaled score of 494 being obtained.

Case 2 (Bill)

Case 2 (Bill), aged 7;2 at the time of tumour diagnosis. He underwent subtotal resection of a medulloblastoma and the insertion of a ventricular drain. Immediately post-surgery, Bill spoke clearly, followed commands and exhibited facial symmetry.

Four days post-surgery, raised pressure in the posterior fossa was detected by CT. Consequently, Bill underwent two further operations, the first to remove the right ventricular drain which had become ineffective, and the second, performed 24 hours later, to insert a left external ventricular drain. Bill experienced a small intracerebral haemorrhage at the site of the original ventricular drain. His mental state deteriorated over the ensuing 12 hours but improved following the positioning of the replacement drain. A CT scan obtained 1 week later revealed a satisfactory reduction in ventricular size. The perilesional haematoma had been partially reabsorbed and there was less mass effect in the posterior fossa. One month after tumour removal, a 6-week course of radiotherapy was initiated.

At all four assessments, Bill presented as a quiet, very co-operative boy who attended well to every task presented. The results of the TOLD-P, administered at the first three assessments, and the TOLD-I, employed at the fourth language evaluation, are shown in Table 4.3. Ten weeks post-surgery, Bill's overall Spoken Language Quotient was within normal limits, however, poorer performances on listening and semantic tasks were recorded. Word-finding difficulties were also observed during test and play situations. Bill's average Spoken Language Quotient was no doubt maintained by the average and above average Speaking and Syntax Quotients obtained. These quotients reflect Bill's outstanding performance on the Sentence Imitation subtest (see Table 4.3). Bill's sentence repetitions appeared echolalic in nature. This observation is supported by the fact that Bill's Sentence Imitation score dropped markedly by the third assessment while his Spoken Language Quotient was maintained (see Table 4.3).

Table 4.3 Case 2 (Bill): Language quotients and subtest standard scores obtained on the *Test of Language Development* — *Primary* (TOLD-P) and the *Test of Language Development* — *Intermediate* (TOLD-I)

TOLD-P	Time post-surgery	SLQ	LiQ	SpQ	SeQ	SyQ	PV	OV	GU	SI	GC
1	10 weeks	98	85	109	73*	117	6*	5*	9	17	12
2	8.5 months	104	88	115	97	109	10	9	6*	17	11
3	15 months	104	100	106	106	102	13	9	7	12	12

TOLD-I	Time post-surgery	SLQ	LiQ	SpQ	SeQ	SyQ	SC	Ch	WO	Gen	GCo
4	28 months	96	97	96	103	91	8	10	9	11	9

Note: Quotients: mean = 100, SD = 15; subtest standard scores: mean = 10, SD = 3. SLQ = Spoken Language Quotient; LiQ = Listening Quotient; SpQ = Speaking Quotient; SeQ = Semantics Quotient; SyQ = Syntax Quotient; PV = Picture Vocabulary Subtest; OV = Oral Vocabulary Subtest; GU = Grammatic Understanding Subtest; SI = Sentence Imitation Subtest; GC = Grammatic Completion Subtest; SC = Sentence Combining Subtest; Ch = Characteristics Subtest; WO = Word Ordering subtest; Gen = Generals Subtest; GCo = Grammatic Comprehension Subtest.
* Below average result (from Hudson and Murdoch, 1992a).

At the time of the second language evaluation, Bill had returned to his Grade 2 class, however, it had been decided that he would repeat Grade 2 the following year. A slight improvement in his overall language abilities was recorded (see Table 4.3). In particular, increased Listening and Semantics Quotients meant that all of the language areas evaluated were well within normal limits on this test. A neuropsychologist also determined normal intelligence quotients (IQ) at this time with scores of 110 (Full Scale IQ), 118 (Verbal IQ) and 100 (Performance IQ) being obtained.

The third language evaluation showed that Bill had maintained his level of language functioning (see Table 4.3). In addition, the peaks and troughs previously recorded for specific language areas had stabilized, resulting in similar quotients being obtained for listening, speaking, semantics and syntax. Although Bill's Speaking and Syntax Quotients declined over the 13 months that elapsed since the completion of treatment, they were still within the normal range at the time of the third assessment. It is speculated that the declines in the Speaking and Syntax Quotients are due to the resolution of the echolalia that may have initially affected the Sentence Imitation score.

Twelve months elapsed between the third and fourth assessments due to a family transfer. Bill was then aged 9;6, hence, the TOLD-I was administered. Bill's language quotients dropped slightly (see Table 4.3) suggesting that he was not as competent at completing more advanced language subtests. However, his language skills were still within the average range for the TOLD-I.

Bill maintained an average level of performance on the BNT at all four assessments, despite the word-finding difficulty noted 10 weeks post-surgery.

Finally, administration of the *Token Test for Children*, 13 months after the completion of treatment, resulted in Bill obtaining a scaled score of 503, which is indicative of an average level of language comprehension.

Thus, overall, Bill demonstrated marginal gains in his level of language functioning during the 13 months since completing a course of radiotherapy for the treatment of a posterior fossa medulloblastoma.

Case 3 (Joe)

At the age of 5;9, Case 3 (Joe) underwent the surgical insertion of a right VP shunt and the total excision of a medulloblastoma.

The results of the TOLD-P are detailed in Table 4.4. At the initial evaluation, Joe presented as an alert, co-operative boy who had just returned to his Grade 1 class after having missed two months of the school year. He obtained a Spoken Language Quotient within average range and performed within normal limits in the areas of listening, speaking and syntax but achieved a below average Semantics Quotient.

Six months after the initial language evaluation, Joe's Grade 1 teacher was satisfied with his progress, however, his mother expressed some concerns. During the second assessment, Joe was quiet and withdrawn. He avoided eye contact and rarely spoke in full sentences. Although his manner was pleasant and co-operative, his attention often had to be directed back to the assessment task. These behavioural characteristics contrasted markedly with Joe's presentation at the first assessment. Most of the language quotients obtained on the second administration of the TOLD-P fell below the initial results reported (see Table 4.4), the only improvements being Joe's semantic and listening abilities.

Table 4.4 Case 3 (Joe): Language quotients and subtest standard scores obtained on the *Test of Language Development — Primary* (TOLD-P)

Test	Time post-surgery	SLQ	LiQ	SpQ	SeQ	SyQ	PV	OV	GU	SI	GC
1	11 weeks	98	91	104	82*	111	6*	8	11	13	11
2	9 months	86	94	83*	94	83*	11	7	7	9	6*
3	17 months	82*	88	81*	88	81*	10	6*	6*	6*	9

Note: Quotients: mean = 100, SD = 15; subtest standard scores: mean = 10, SD = 3. SLQ = Spoken Language Quotient; LiQ = Listening Quotient; SpQ = Speaking Quotient; SeQ = Semantics Quotient; SyQ = Syntax Quotient; PV = Picture Vocabulary Subtest; OV = Oral Vocabulary Subtest; GU = Grammatic Understanding Subtest; SI = Sentence Imitation Subtest; GC = Grammatic Completion Subtest.
* Below average result (from Hudson and Murdoch, 1992a).

When the third post-surgery language assessment was attempted, Joe exhibited extreme distress and refused to become involved in any activity that was presented. Joe's mother reported that he was becoming increasingly afraid of failing any school activities. Consequently, two sessions were spent regaining Joe's confidence. The assessments were then completed in a relaxed, enjoyable manner in the surrounds of his own home.

A further reduction in language quotients was recorded at the third assessment (see Table 4.4). Below average Spoken Language, Speaking and Syntax Quotients were obtained. Previous Spoken Language Quotients were within the normal range of 85–115. Although Joe's Semantics Quotient declined, it was still in advance of the semantic abilities recorded one month post-treatment. Examination of specific subtests revealed Joe's use of morphological endings to be the only area of improvement. Although the TOLD-P results suggest that Joe's language abilities were deteriorating, closer examination of the subtest raw scores obtained at each of the three assessments implied that Joe's language skills had at least been maintained and perhaps even advanced a little. This being the case, the deterioration indicated by the language quotients and standard scores (see Table 4.4) would reflect limited language advancement relative to that of his peers.

An improvement in expressive vocabulary was recorded across the first two administrations of the BNT. Joe's score increased from 23 correct responses out of a possible 60 to 31 correct responses. A score of 27 was attained at the third assessment. At this time (15 months post-treatment), semantic and phonemic paraphasias and non-words were prominent throughout the BNT and in conversational speech. Residual word-finding difficulties were also noted.

The *Token Test for Children* which was administered 14 months post-treatment revealed a scaled score 487 which is below average. An increasing number of errors were made when the instructions involved more than one adjective qualifying the token to be selected (e.g. small, yellow circle), prepositions and clauses.

Thus, apart from semantic abilities, a decline in language competency was recorded during the 14 months following the completion of CNS irradiation. It is possible that Joe's behaviour at the time of the second language evaluation was related to his reduced language scores, however, despite the optimum test behaviour at the time of the final assessment session, a further reduction in language scores was recorded.

Factors influencing language recovery in children treated for brain tumours

The changes in language abilities documented in the three cases described above indicate that the pattern of language recovery exhibited by children following surgical excision and irradiation of a posterior fossa medulloblastoma is variable. Although one subject (Case 1 — Jane) demonstrated marginal improvements in her language function over a 19-month period post-radiotherapy, her language abilities remained below the average range expected for a child of her age. In contrast, all aspects of the language abilities of another subject (Case 2 — Bill) were at an age-appropriate level six months after the completion of radiotherapy. Case 3 (Joe), exhibited a pattern of language change that differed to both of the above subjects, showing a decline in language abilities during the first 14 months post-treatment. In that all three subjects underwent a similar surgical procedure and were exposed to a similar level of radiation, it is difficult to provide any simple explanation for the degree of variation observed in their language abilities. It is possible that individuals vary widely in their vulnerability to the effects of radiotherapy or that subtle differences in the surgical procedure have important consequences for the later functioning of the CNS. With regard to the latter explanation, however, it is of interest to note that the subject who appeared to experience the greatest number of post-surgical complications (i.e. Case 2 — Bill) also exhibited the least impaired language abilities.

The age at which each case was diagnosed and treated may also have contributed to the varying outcomes. It has been proposed that children treated for posterior fossa tumour when less than six years of age are at risk of deteriorating in the long term (Danoff et al., 1982; Mulhern and Kun, 1985). This may explain the deteriorating language scores exhibited by Case 3, however, the language deficits experienced by Case 1 also persisted despite Case 1 being aged 10;6 at the time of treatment. Thus, an interruption to the developmental acquisition of language skills is not the only factor contributing to the communication deficits experienced by children treated for posterior fossa tumours.

Although all three subjects demonstrated below average semantic quotients on either the TOLD-P or TOLD-I when initially assessed, all demonstrated considerable improvements in their semantic abilities during the first six months after treatment. Semantic gains and a reduction in the number of semantic and phonemic paraphasias were also indicated by the BNT. Residual word-finding difficulties, however, were still evident during the final assessment sessions. Brouwers et al. (1985) detected word-finding difficulties in 13 of 23 children treated with radiotherapy and chemotherapy for leukaemia. They claimed that such a deficit could be related to poor semantic knowledge, as in cases of posterior temporal damage, or to a lack of verbal spontaneity, as seen in patients with frontal lobe abnormalities. Whereas the presence of semantic–lexical deficits in children exposed to CNS prophylaxis has been recognized by a number of authors (Painter et al., 1975; Brouwers et al., 1985; Taylor et al., 1987; Hudson et al., 1989), few, if any, studies have documented the recovery of such deficits.

The infratentorial location of the tumours removed from the three subjects described above suggests that any long-term post-surgical disturbances observed, such as in Cases 1 (Jane) and 3 (Joe) are likely to be the result of either structural damage to the cerebrum caused by exposure to radiation as part of the course of radiotherapy or complications of the surgery itself which influence the functioning of the cerebrum in some secondary manner. As none of the three subjects examined had any language impairment evident before surgery, it appears that the language disturbances observed post-treatment can not be attributed to the direct effects of the tumour itself. This observation is further supported by the absence of recurrent or residual tumour in all three subjects throughout the duration of the study. All three subjects did, however, experience hydrocephalus requiring the surgical insertion of VP shunts. Although it is possible that the raised intracranial pressure may have caused some compression of the cerebrum, and thereby influenced the language abilities of the subjects in the short term, it is unlikely to be the cause of the long-term language problems exhibited by Cases 1 (Jane) and 3 (Joe).

Kun et al. (1983) examined the intellectual abilities of 30 children immediately after they were irradiated for brain tumours and found that the presence of increased intracranial pressure did not differentiate between those exhibiting intellectual deficits and those whose level of intelligence was within normal limits. This is supported by the finding of Hudson and Murdoch (1992a) that although Case 2 (Bill) experienced elevated intracranial pressure post-surgery, as the result of a failed ventricular drain, his language abilities were the least impaired of the three subjects investigated.

Structural and functional changes in the cerebrum resulting from exposure to radiation during radiotherapy would appear, therefore, to offer the best explanation for the presence of long-term disturbances in the language abilities of Case 1 (Jane). In that it has been reported that structural changes in the brain such as calcification, necrosis and atrophy may occur up to 48 years post-radiotherapy (Lee and Suh, 1977; Pearson et al., 1983; Lichtor et al., 1984; Curnes et al., 1986), it is possible that although having shown some recovery over the 28-month period to date, the language abilities of Case 1 (Jane) could decline at some later stage. In addition, it is also possible that, although normal at present, the language abilities of Case 2 (Bill) may also decline in future years. There is a need, therefore, for even longer-term studies to investigate the effects of cancer treatment on language.

In summary, the language profiles, documented in the present chapter, of three children who experienced surgery and CNS irradiation for the treatment of posterior fossa medulloblastoma indicated that such treatment has variable effects on language ability in the period up to 28 months post-treatment. Further, although severe semantic–lexical deficits may be present immediately post-treatment, in all three cases reported, semantic abilities improved dramatically within the first six months after treatment.

References

Alajouanine T, Lhermitte, F (1965) Acquired aphasia in children. Brain 88: 653–662.

Broadbent VA, Barnes ND, Wheeler TK (1981) Medulloblastoma in childhood: long-term results of treatment. Cancer 48: 26–30.

Brouwers P, Riccardi R, Fedio P, Poplack DG (1985) Long-term neuropsychologic sequelae of childhood leukemia: correlation with CT brain scan abnormalities. Journal of Pediatrics 106: 723–728.

Carrow-Woolfolk E, Lynch J (1982) An Integrated Approach to Language Disorders in Children. Orlando, FL: Grune & Stratton.

Curnes JT, Laster DW, Ball MR, Moody DM, Witcofski RL (1986) MRI of radiation injury to the brain. American Journal of Roentgenology 147: 119–124.

Danoff BF, Chowchock FS, Marquette C, Mulgrew L, Kramer S (1982) Assessment of the long-term effects of primary radiation therapy for brain tumours in children. Cancer 49: 1580–1586.

Davis PC, Hoffman JC, Pearl GS, Braun IF (1986) CT evaluation of effects of cranial radiation therapy in children. American Journal of Roentgenology 147: 587–592.

De Reuck J, vander Eecken, H (1975) The anatomy of the late radiation encephalopathy. European Neurology 13: 481–494.

DiSimoni F (1978) The Token Test for Children. Hingham, MA: Teaching Resources.

Dooms GC, Hecht S, Brant-Zawadzki M, Berthiaume Y, Norman D, Newton TH (1986) Brain radiation lesions: MR imaging. Radiology 158: 149–155.

Duffner PK, Cohen ME, Thomas RM, Lansky SB (1985) The long-term effects of cranial irradiation on the central nervous system. Cancer 56: 1841–1846.

Hammill DD, Newcomer PL (1982) Test of Language Development — Intermediate. Austin, TX: Pro-Ed.

Hudson LJ, Murdoch BE (1992a) Language recovery following surgery and CNS prophylaxis for the treatment of childhood medulloblastoma: a prospective study of three cases. Aphasiology 6: 17–28.

Hudson LJ, Murdoch BE (1992b) Chronic language deficits in children treated for posterior fossa tumour. Aphasiology 6: 135–150.

Hudson LJ, Murdoch BE, Ozanne AE (1989) Posterior fossa tumours in childhood: associated speech and language disorders post-surgery. Aphasiology 3: 1–18.

Kaplan E, Goodglass H, Weintraub S (1983) Boston Naming Test. Philadelphia, PA: Lea & Febiger.

Kun LE, Mulhern RK, Crisco JJ (1983) Quality of life in children treated for brain tumour. Journal of Neurosurgery 58: 1–6.

Lee KF, Suh JH (1977) CT evidence of grey matter calcification secondary to radiation therapy. Computerized Tomography 1: 103–110.

Lichtor T, Wollman RL, Brown FD (1984) Calcified basal ganglionic mass 12 years after radiation therapy for medulloblastoma. Surgical Neurology 21: 373–376.

Marks JE, Baglan RJ, Prassad SC, Blank WF (1981) Cerebral radionecrosis: incidence and risk in relation to dose, time, fractionation and volume. International Journal of Radiation Oncology, Biology and Physics 7: 243–252.

Mulhern RK, Kun LE (1985) Neuropsychologic function in children with brain tumours: III. Interval changes in the six months following treatment. Medical and Pediatric Oncology 13: 318–324.

Murdoch BE, Hudson-Tennent LJ (1994) Differential language outcomes in children following treatment for posterior fossa tumours. Aphasiology 8: 507–534.

Newcomer PL, Hammill DD (1982) Test of Language Development — Primary. Austin, TX: Pro-Ed.

Packer RJ, Sutton LN, Atkins TE, Radcliffe J, Bunin GR, D'Angio G, Siegel KR, Schut L (1989) A prospective study of cognitive function in children receiving whole-brain radiotherapy and chemotherapy: 2-year results. Journal of Neurosurgery 70: 707–713.

Painter MJ, Chutorian AM, Hilal SK (1975) Cerebrovasculopathy following irradiation in childhood. Neurology 25: 189–194.

Pearson ADJ, Campbell AN, McAllister VL, Pearson GL (1983) Intracranial calcification in survivors of childhood medulloblastoma. Archives of Disease in Childhood 58: 133–136.

Price DB, Hotson GC, Loh JP (1988) Pontine calcification following radiotherapy: CT demonstration. Journal of Computed Assisted Tomography 12: 45–46.

Satz P, Bullard-Bates C (1981) Acquired aphasia in children. In Sarno MT (ed.) Acquired Aphasia. New York: Academic Press, 398–426.

Silverman CL, Palkes H, Talent B, Kovnar E, Clouse JW, Thomas PRM (1984) Late effects of radiotherapy on patients with cerebellar medulloblastoma. Cancer 54: 825–829.

Taylor HG, Albo VC, Phebus CK, Sachs BR, Bierl PG (1987) Post-irradiation treatment outcomes for children with acute lymphocytic leukaemia: clarification of risks. Journal of Pediatric Psychology 12: 395–411.

Tsuruda JS, Kortman KE, Bradley WG, Wheeler DC, Van Dalsem W, Bradley TP (1987) Radiation effects on cerebral white matter: MR evaluation. American Journal of Roentgenology 149: 165–171.

Van Dongen HR, Loonen MCB (1977) Factors related to prognosis of acquired aphasia in children. Cortex 13: 131–136.

Wright TL, Bresnan MJ (1976) Radiation induced cerebrovascular disease in children. Neurology 26: 540–543.

Chapter 5
Variability in patterns of language impairment in children following treatment for posterior fossa tumour

BRUCE E MURDOCH AND LISA J HUDSON

Introduction

When considered as a group, the language abilities of children treated for posterior fossa tumours have been reported to be less competent than those of normal children of the same age and sex (Hudson and Murdoch, 1992) (see Chapter 3). With the exception of confrontation naming, rapid naming, word fluency and reading and writing abilities, most of the areas of language tested by Hudson and Murdoch (1992) were found to be impaired in children treated for tumours compared to their age- and sex-matched peers. Closer examination of the data presented by Hudson and Murdoch (1992), however, reveals that not only did the overall language abilities of the tumour patients vary considerably from individual to individual (some children exhibited a significant language disorder while others had apparently normal language abilities) but also performance of the tumour subjects on specific language tasks varied widely. This variation might be attributed to any one or a combination of variables including tumour type, surgical complications, age, the need for radiotherapy, presence or absence of hydrocephalus, etc. (see Chapter 2). Consequently, it was thought by Murdoch and Hudson-Tennent (1994) that by presenting their data on a group basis only, Hudson and Murdoch (1992) had missed important information concerning the variety of language outcomes following treatment for posterior fossa tumour.

Based on the premise that better insight into the language abilities of children treated for posterior fossa tumours could be gained by examining each case on an individual basis, Murdoch and Hudson-Tennent (1994) re-examined the language findings of the same 20

89

children treated for posterior fossa tumour reported by Hudson and Murdoch (1992). To demonstrate the variability in language outcome following treatment for brain tumour and to enable any observed language problem to be described and discussed with reference to individual variables relating to personal details, medical conditions and treatment factors, the 20 cases reported by Murdoch and Hudson-Tennent (1994) are outlined below. Relevant medical and biographical details for the 20 children reported are listed in Table 3.1 in Chapter 3.

The language test battery administered included the age-appropriate test from the *Test of Language Development* (TOLD) series, the *Token Test for Children* (DiSimoni, 1978), Subtests 7, 8 and 9 of the *Clinical Evaluation of Language Functions* (CELF) (Semel and Wiig, 1982), the *Boston Naming Test* (BNT) (Kaplan et al., 1983) and the *Test of Language Competence* (TLC) (Wiig and Secord, 1985). According to each subject's age, the test administered from the TOLD series was either:

- *Test of Language Development — Primary* (TOLD-P) (Newcomer and Hammill, 1982) (age range 4;0–8;11).
- *Test of Language Development — Intermediate* (TOLD-I) (Hammill and Newcomer, 1982) (age range 8;6–12;11).
- *Test of Adolescent Language 2* (TOAL-2) (Hammill et al., 1987) (age range 12;0–18;5).

For further details of the language tests see Chapter 3.

Case reports

Case 1 (Robert)

Robert underwent total excision of a fourth ventricle ependymoma at the age of 3 years. Despite evidence of hydrocephalus pre-surgery, a ventriculoperitoneal (VP) shunt was not required. Instead, a right external ventricular drain was inserted during surgery and remained in place for 5 days. Robert made a rapid recovery and was discharged from hospital 7 days post-surgery. A 6-week course of craniospinal irradiation was administered, involving a tumour dose of 5000 rads delivered in 31 fractions, whole brain irradiation of 4000 rads (25 fractions) and 3200 rads (20 fractions) delivered to the spine.

A speech and language evaluation was performed one year five months post-surgery when Robert was aged 4;5. At that time Robert presented as a talkative, outgoing child, characteristics which, according to his mother, developed quickly following tumour treatment. No other behavioural changes were reported to have occurred post-treatment.

TOLD-P

Robert achieved an Overall Language Quotient of 89 which is within the test's normal range of 85–115. Closer examination of Robert's test performance revealed average abilities in the areas of expressive semantics and syntax, but below average receptive abilities. Standard scores of 6 (below average) on the Picture Vocabulary and Grammatic Understanding subtests of the TOLD-P were obtained. Both of these subtests require the subject to select the appropriate picture in response to a word or sentence provided by the examiner. The Picture Vocabulary and Grammatic Understanding scores converted into a below average Listening Quotient of 76. A Speaking Quotient of 100 indicated a marked discrepancy between Robert's expressive and receptive language abilities.

Token Test for Children

The reduction in receptive language abilities demonstrated by Robert on the TOLD-P was also evident on the *Token Test for Children*. Robert obtained an Overall Age Scaled Score of 492 (Token Test Mean = 500 ± 5). It was noted that while he could identify colours and shapes, he was unable to name them spontaneously. A lack of consolidated knowledge may account for the below average scores obtained by Robert on this test. The *Token Test for Children* involves attention and auditory memory skills as well as language comprehension abilities. Robert's performance on this test suggests that memory and attentional deficits cannot account for the marked comprehension deficit detected by the TOLD-P.

CELF

Robert was unable to attempt Subtest 7 (Producing Word Series) and Subtest 8 (Producing Names on Confrontation) of the CELF as he could not name the days of the week, months of the year, colours, or shapes. He reached criterion on Subtest 9, Producing Word Associations (i.e. word fluency).

BNT

Fourteen of the 60 test items were correctly named. Normative data, however, is not available for four-year-old children. Stimulus and phonemic cues did not assist Robert's performance.

Summary of language abilities

Robert presented with a receptive language deficit. Although he was able to follow many of the oral commands given in the *Token Test for Children*, Robert's performance deteriorated when attempting the TOLD-P comprehension tasks. Although these subtests include shorter test items than the *Token Test for Children*, they are more complex semantically and syntactically.

Case 2 (Roxanne)

At the age of 3;2 Roxanne was admitted to hospital for the investigation of a 5-week history of headaches, vomiting and ataxia. During this time a marked deterioration in the clarity of Roxanne's speech was also reported by her parents. At the time of hospital admission, Roxanne's speech was described by her parents as 'almost unintelligible' and 'very nasal'. A CT scan performed on admission revealed the presence of a left posterior fossa tumour, which appeared cystic in nature. A left craniotomy was performed and the tumour partially excised. Diagnosis was that of a low-grade, pilocytic, juvenile astrocytoma. Roxanne was able to speak immediately following surgery, however, 8 days post-surgery nursing staff observed excessively nasal speech. A speech therapy referral was requested but not acted upon. Twelve days post-surgery a VP shunt was inserted to alleviate persisting hydrocephalus. Roxanne experienced an uneventful post-operative recovery. According to her parents, improvement in Roxanne's speech was minimal. She commenced a course of radiotherapy 1 month post-surgery.

At the time of language assessment, at age 5;10, Roxanne presented as an energetic, outgoing girl who completed all test procedures with interest and enthusiasm.

TOLD-P

Administration of the TOLD-P yielded an Overall Language Quotient of 89 which falls within the test's average range of 85–115. Roxanne's listening, speaking, and syntactic abilities also fell within normal limits as determined by the TOLD-P. Semantic abilities were shown to be below average with a quotient of 82 being obtained. This was due to a below average result on the Picture Vocabulary (receptive) Subtest. Expressive vocabulary, as assessed by the Oral Vocabulary Subtest, was shown to be within normal limits. The standard score obtained for expressive syntax (Sentence Imitation Subtest) was below average which contrasts with the sound performance recorded for the receptive syntax (Grammatic Understanding) task.

It was noted that although Roxanne performed within the normal range on the Grammatic Completion Subtest of the TOLD-P, she tended to omit morphological endings during conversational speech. This suggests that while Roxanne's phonological system does not consistently permit the production of word endings, she has incorporated morphemes into her language knowledge base.

Token Test for Children

Roxanne obtained a below average Overall Age Scaled Score of 490. She experienced increasing difficulty as the length of the commands increased, frequently confusing the first colour or shape specified in the command with the second colour or shape mentioned (e.g. she selected the green circle and red square instead of the green square and red circle). In Part V, Roxanne comprehended 14 of the 21 concepts presented. Concepts which led to confusion included *except, together, quickly/slowly, between, after* and *before*. Other errors in Part V resulted from a failure to manipulate the correct tokens.

CELF

Roxanne performed above criterion on Subtests 7, 8 and 9 of the CELF.

BNT

A score of 19 on the BNT was just below the normal range of 20–37 specified by the test's normative data for a child of Roxanne's age.

Summary of language abilities

Roxanne exhibited language deficits in the areas of receptive semantics, expressive syntax and word-finding abilities. Although Roxanne was able to select the correct pictures in the Grammatic Understanding Subtest of the TOLD-P, she demonstrated difficulty following the *Token Test for Children* commands. The forced alternative format and the visual stimuli provided by the TOLD-P may have assisted Roxanne's syntactic comprehension during this test.

Case 3 (Roger)

Roger was hospitalized at the age of 3;10 following a 2-week period of impaired balance, irritability and mild weight loss. A neurological examination indicated bilateral papilloedema and inco-ordination to be the only abnormalities. A CT scan performed on admission revealed moderate hydrocephalus with dilatation of the third and lateral ventricles associated with a mass lesion in the foramen magnum and fourth ventricle. A posterior fossa craniotomy was performed resulting in the total removal of the medulloblastoma. A right external ventricular drain was inserted during surgery, however, continued high cerebrospinal fluid (CSF) pressure resulted in the drain being replaced by a VP shunt 7 days after the initial surgery. Roger then experienced a rapid, uneventful recovery. Roger underwent a course of radiotherapy to the whole brain and spinal cord. A CT scan performed 22 months post-operatively showed the presence of calcification in the pons, temporal lobes and posterior temporal regions and in the white matter of the frontal lobes. These areas of calcification were attributed to the CNS irradiation experienced by Roger. There was no evidence of tumour recurrence at this time.

On assessment two years five months post-surgery, Roger presented as an alert, co-operative six-year-old child who was still attending pre-school as his teacher believed he was not yet able to cope in a Grade 1 class. Two and a half years post-surgery, Roger experienced a fourth ventricle haemorrhage and a left temporo-parietal infarct. A VP shunt revision and prolonged hospitalization followed. Roger was then admitted to a paediatric rehabilitation centre to permit the implementation of intensive therapy programmes. Testing by Murdoch and Hudson-Tennent (1994) ceased at that time. Consequently the *Token Test for Children* and the BNT were not administered to Roger.

TOLD-P

Roger obtained a below average Overall Spoken Language Quotient of 81 and below average quotients for Speaking (expressive language) and Syntax (expressive and receptive). Performance on specific subtests of the TOLD-P included below average scores for Oral Vocabulary (expressive semantics), Grammatic Understanding (syntactic comprehension), and Sentence Imitation (expressive syntax). The Grammatic Completion (morphology) subtest score was in the low–average range.

CELF

Roger did not know the days of the week in order to complete Subtest 7 (Producing Word Series) and hence scored below criterion on this task. He produced 33 correct responses out of a possible 36 on Subtest 8 (Producing Names on Confrontation), which is within the test's normal range. The number of words produced in Subtest 9 (Producing Word Associations) was well within normal limits indicating intact word fluency ability.

Summary of language abilities

Roger demonstrated deficits in all language areas except receptive vocabulary and morphology. Structural damage to the CNS was documented by CT and may have contributed to Roger's language impairment. Although the effects of cerebral calcification on language functions have not been determined, intellectual, concentration and academic impairments have been identified in children with evidence of CNS calcification (Hodges and Smithells, 1983; Pearson et al., 1983).

Case 4 (Jacinta)

At the age of 5;1, Jacinta underwent investigations for a 1-month history of vomiting, headaches and transient incidences of slurred speech. A CT scan revealed the presence of a 5-cm mass in the right cerebellar hemisphere extending across the midline and involving the vermis (see Figure 5.1). The fourth ventricle was displaced to the left and anteriorly and high-grade obstructive hydrocephalus was observed. Jacinta underwent the total excision of a large cerebellar astrocytoma and subsequently experienced a rapid, uneventful recovery. No further treatments, including radiotherapy, were required.

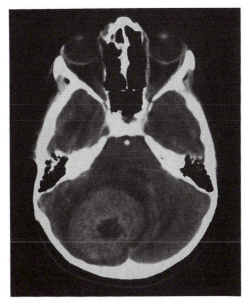

Figure 5.1: Case 4 (Jacinta): Pre-operative CT scan showing a 5-cm mass in the right cerebellar hemisphere extending across the midline.

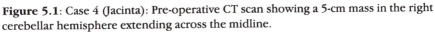

Language assessments were performed one year two months post-surgery. At this time Jacinta was aged 6;3, and was succeeding in Grade 1 as well as at extra-curricular activities such as piano and ballet classes.

TOLD-P

Jacinta obtained above average quotients on all of the language areas assessed by the TOLD-P.

Token Test for Children

An Overall Age Scaled Score of 506 was achieved on the *Token Test for Children*. This is slightly above the test's average range of 495–505.

CELF

Jacinta performed above criterion on Subtests, 7, 8 and 9 of the CELF.

BNT

Jacinta achieved a score of 47 out of a possible 60 items on the BNT. This is above the range of 20–34 (mean = 29) obtained by the Grade 1 children assessed by Kaplan et al. (1983).

Summary of language abilities

Jacinta achieved above average language scores on the tests administered.

Case 5 (Morris)

Morris was admitted to hospital at the age of 5;9 due to a 2-month history of unsteady gait and a 1-month history of headaches and nausea. Ataxia and horizontal nystagmus were the only neurological abnormalities evident on examination. A CT scan performed on admission demonstrated the presence of a large midline posterior fossa mass which was displacing the fourth ventricle upwards and to the right, and causing marked hydrocephalus and some periventricular oedema. A right VP shunt was inserted to alleviate the hydrocephalus and 5 days later a medulloblastoma, 5 cm in diameter, was totally resected. Morris recovered rapidly and was discharged from hospital 9 days after tumour removal. Two weeks later, Morris commenced a course of radiotherapy which involved a total dose of 4800 rads delivered in 30 fractions to the whole brain and spinal cord.

Morris was tested by Murdoch and Hudson-Tennent (1994) when aged 7;1. At this time he was in a normal Grade 2 class but was experiencing some difficulties with mathematics and reading. He presented as a withdrawn child, who, according to his mother, was anxious about failing any school-related tasks.

TOLD-P

An Overall Language Quotient of 82 (below average) was obtained by Morris. Below average quotients were also recorded in the areas of expressive language (Speaking Quotient) and expressive and receptive syntax (Syntax Quotient). Receptive language and semantic abilities were in the low–average range on the TOLD-P. The TOLD-P subtests indicated that Morris experienced particular difficulty with Oral Vocabulary (expressive semantics), Grammatic Understanding (syntactic comprehension), and Sentence Imitation (expressive syntax). Picture Vocabulary (receptive semantics) and Grammatic Completion (morphology) scores were within normal limits.

Token Test for Children

Morris experienced increasing difficulty on the *Token Test for Children* as the instructions increased in length and complexity. His Overall Age Scaled Score of 491 was greater than 1 SD below the test's mean of 500.

This result concurs with Morris' performance on the Grammatic Understanding Subtest of the TOLD-P where an increase in complexity (but not length) resulted in an increase in errors.

CELF

For Subtest 7 (Producing Word Series), Morris named six of the seven week days, which is below criterion for a Grade 2 child. He was unable to label the colours and shapes in Subtest 8 (Producing Names on Confrontation) and, hence, scored below criterion on this task. Word fluency (Subtest 9, Producing Word Associations) was within normal limits, however, three incidences of perseveration were recorded during this task.

BNT

Morris scored 26 out of 60 on the BNT, which was below normal according to the test norms.

Summary of language abilities

Impairments in syntactic comprehension and expression, and expressive vocabulary were exhibited by Morris. Although his lack of confidence may have influenced his test performance, it may also be postulated that his anxiety towards school work was caused by his inability to cope with the language demands placed on him in an educational setting. Increasing either the length or complexity of syntactic structures resulted in Morris making a greater number of errors.

Case 6 (Pamela)

Pamela was admitted to hospital at the age of 3;2 for the investigation of a 3-week history of papilloedema and an unsteady, wide-based gait. A CT scan indicated the presence of a partly cystic, soft tissue mass just to the left of the midline in the posterior fossa. The tumour measured 4.5 cm in diameter and was displacing the fourth ventricle laterally to the right. Resultant obstructive hydrocephalus was observed with dilation of the third and lateral ventricles. A right VP shunt was inserted to relieve the hydrocephalus and 4 days later a posterior fossa craniotomy was performed. A juvenile pilocytic astrocytoma was subtotally removed. Pamela was discharged from hospital 2 weeks after tumour resection and continued to make a steady, uneventful recovery. No further treatments, including radiotherapy, were required.

Pamela's language abilities were assessed at four years two months post-surgery when she was aged 7;4. At this time, she was a Grade 2 student in a multi-age Grade 1 and 2 combined class and was receiving eight hours individual tuition each week. She had just been accepted into a small remedial class. Pamela presented as an enthusiastic, talkative child who enjoyed the assessment tasks presented to her over three testing sessions.

TOLD-P

Pamela scored an Overall Language Quotient of 74, which was below the average range of 85–115 provided by the TOLD-P. Closer examination of Pamela's TOLD-P results indicated that her expressive language skills were in advance of her receptive language abilities. Her Listening Quotient of 64 was greater than 2 SD below the test's mean of 100. This score resulted from poor performances on the Picture Vocabulary and Grammatic Understanding subtests of the TOLD-P. Pamela demonstrated difficulty comprehending the verb tenses and negative structures included in the Grammatic Understanding Subtest. Only Pamela's Speaking Quotient (i.e. expressive semantics and syntax) fell within the test's normal range. The Semantics and Syntax Quotients obtained by Pamela were below average due to her below average receptive Subtest scores and borderline expressive results. It was noted during testing that Pamela did not have difficulty remembering the test instructions or sentences, and could often repeat them or correct her response two test items later. This finding suggested the presence of a slowed language processing ability.

Token Test for Children

Pamela experienced no difficulty completing Parts I to IV of the *Token Test for Children*, however, her performance deteriorated during Part V when concepts and dependent clauses were introduced. Pamela frequently used repetition of the instruction as a strategy, but still manipulated the tokens incorrectly.

As observed during administration of the TOLD-P, Pamela was able to remember the instructions, irrespective of their length, but failed to process complex structures and concepts.

CELF

Pamela performed within normal limits on Subtests 7, 8 and 9 of the CELF.

BNT

Pamela achieved a low score of 16 on the BNT, a score markedly below the normal range of 34–45 specified by the test norms.

Summary of language abilities

Pamela exhibited a generalized language impairment with particular difficulties being evident on receptive language tasks. Expressive skills were shown to be at a borderline level. It is noteworthy that language impairments were evident despite an absence of CNS prophylaxis in Pamela's medical history.

Case 7 (Joseph)

Joseph was diagnosed with a posterior fossa tumour at the age of 21 months following a 3-month history of ataxia and tilting his head to the right. A suboccipital craniotomy was performed but only tumour biopsy was possible. Diagnosis was that of a Grade I/II solid astrocytoma. Two weeks post-surgery a right VP shunt was inserted. Further surgery was required one week later to reposition the shunt. Five weeks following tumour biopsy a 4-week course of radiotherapy was initiated. A CT scan obtained at the conclusion of CNS irradiation showed no evidence of residual or recurrent tumour or of increased intracranial pressure. Four and a half months post-irradiation, a CT scan demonstrated the presence of a small lesion slightly to the left of the midline in the posterior fossa. This was thought to be recurrent tumour. At the time of the language assessment, performed 5 years 8 months post-surgery, this condition had not changed.

Joseph was aged 7;5 when administered the language test battery. He exhibited a severe sensorineural hearing loss in his left ear but normal hearing in his right ear. Joseph's hearing loss was attributed to radiation-induced damage. He was enrolled in a normal Grade 2 class but was experiencing difficulties in all academic areas. He was receiving remedial intervention for reading and spelling. Joseph also exhibited gross and fine motor deficits.

TOLD-P

Joseph's language skills were below average, as indicated by an Overall Language Quotient of 77. Most difficulty was experienced on the semantic subtests of the TOLD-P resulting in a Semantics Quotient of 70, which is 2 SD below the test's mean of 100. Joseph's receptive language abilities were in advance of his expressive language skills. A Speaking Quotient of 74 resulted from poor performances on the Oral Vocabulary, Sentence Imitation and Grammatic Completion Subtests. A sound performance on the Grammatic Understanding Subtest indicated intact syntactic comprehension abilities and resulted in a borderline Listening Quotient of 85 being obtained.

Token Test for Children

Joseph's intact comprehension abilities were confirmed by the ease with which he completed the *Token Test for Children*. He had no difficulty retaining the auditory commands and manipulating the tokens appropriately.

CELF

Joseph's performance on Subtest 7 (Producing Word Series) was below criterion as he was unable to name all seven days of the week correctly. The time taken to complete Subtest 8 (Producing Names on Confrontation) was greater than the 120-second criterion specified by the test. Despite evidence of perseveration, the number of words generated by Joseph on Subtest 9 (Producing Word Associations) was above criterion.

BNT

Joseph correctly named 27 of the 60 BNT items, a score which falls below the test norms for a child of his age.

Summary of language abilities

The language impairments demonstrated by Joseph were in the areas of expressive syntax and receptive and expressive semantics. Auditory comprehension abilities were in advance of his other language skills despite the presence of a severe sensorineural loss in the left ear.

Case 8 (Glen)

At the age of 2;7 Glen underwent investigations for symptoms of ataxia, lethargy and vomiting. Symptoms had been present for 2 to 3 months. A neurological examination revealed bilateral papilloedema and dysfunction of the eighth cranial nerve. A CT scan performed on admission to hospital indicated the presence of a midline tumour arising from the cerebellum. It measured 3.5 cm in anterior–posterior diameter and was associated with obstructive hydrocephalus. A right VP shunt was inserted to alleviate the hydrocephalus, and 5 days later Glen underwent total excision of an ependymoma. Surgery resulted in a marked left facial palsy, which had not resolved at the time of language testing. Glen experienced a particularly slow recovery post-surgery. He spent a prolonged period of 27 days in the hospital's intensive care unit and was reportedly mute for 6 months following tumour removal. He was discharged from hospital 10 weeks post-surgery following a course of radiotherapy, which involved a total dose of 4000 rads to the whole brain and spinal cord. Glen had bilateral grommets inserted at the age of 3;5 to relieve recurrent middle-ear infections. A hearing test performed just prior to the current investigation demonstrated normal hearing sensitivity at all frequencies. Glen's VP shunt required pumping when he was aged 3;8, and shunt revisions were performed when he was aged 5;5 and 6;0. The shunt revisions were required to relieve the presence of hydrocephalus. A CT scan obtained at the time of the final shunt revision showed dramatic ventriculomegaly (abnormal enlargement of the ventricles), which was most marked in the fourth ventricle because of the tumour resection (see Figure 5.2). There was no evidence of tumour recurrence. Glen underwent surgery at the age of 8;3 to correct a left strabismus.

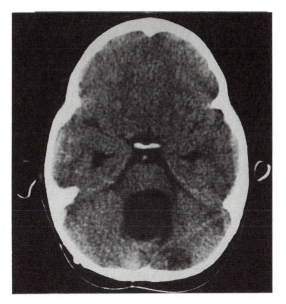

Figure 5.2 Case 8 (Glen): Post-operative CT scan demonstrating dramatic ventriculomegaly, which is most marked in the fourth ventricle due to the tumour resection.

At the time of language assessment Glen was aged 8;8. He presented as a happy, co-operative child who was enjoying Grade 1 at a small country school where he was receiving remedial instruction twice a week. Due to his ataxic gait, he required assistance when walking and wore a helmet to protect his head from frequent falls.

TOLD-P

A severe language delay was indicated by the TOLD-P with all subtests and quotients falling greater than 2 SD below the test's average range.

CELF

Glen was unable to complete Subtests 7 and 8 of the CELF due to an inability to name the required days of the week, colours and shapes. His performance on Subtest 9 (Producing Word Associations) was below criterion.

Summary of language abilities

Glen was severely delayed in all areas of language despite an unremarkable pre-morbid and diagnostic history. Factors which may have contributed to his poor post-treatment language status include the extensive tumour resection experienced, CNS irradiation (although a relatively low dose of 4000 rads was administered), persistent hydro-cephalus and subsequent shunt revisions and recurrent middle-ear infections.

Case 9 (Nigel)

A 2-week history of headache, vomiting and poor concentration preceded the diagnosis of a posterior fossa tumour when Nigel was aged 7;2. A CT scan demonstrated the presence of a left cerebellar hemisphere mass which measured 5 cm in diameter. Hydrocephalus, due to obstruction at the level of the fourth ventricle was also reported. A medulloblastoma was partially excised, and 6 days later a left VP shunt was inserted. Nigel was discharged from hospital 18 days after tumour removal. He then underwent a course of craniospinal irradiation involving a total dose of 5000 rads.

Nigel's language abilities were assessed two years four months post-surgery at the age of 9;6. He was coping in a normal Grade 3 class, after having repeated Grade 2 the previous year.

TOLD-I

Nigel performed within normal limits on all of the TOLD-I measures.

Token Test for Children

Nigel attained average scores on the *Token Test for Children* indicating intact auditory comprehension abilities.

CELF

Nigel performed within normal limits on tasks of rapid language retrieval and production as indicated by the CELF.

BNT

Nigel performed within normal limits on the BNT.

Summary of language abilities

Despite the hydrocephalus, surgery and CNS irradiation experienced, Nigel demonstrated age-appropriate language abilities.

Case 10 (Phillip)

At the age of 7;4, Phillip presented with a two and a half month history of neck stiffness, headaches, vomiting and ataxia. A CT scan indicated the presence of a left cerebellar tumour and an associated increase in intracranial pressure. A juvenile pilocytic astrocytoma (Grade 1) was diagnosed. The tumour was completely excised and Phillip made a rapid recovery. A routine CT scan performed 5 weeks post-surgery revealed residual tumour in the left cerebellar hemisphere. There was no evidence of any mass effect or hydrocephalus. A second suboccipital craniotomy was performed, and a 3-cm cystic astrocytoma was completely removed. Once again, Phillip recovered quickly and was discharged from hospital 5 days after surgery. At this time, Phillip demonstrated a slight gait ataxia not evident after the initial tumour excision.

Phillip's language abilities were assessed at age 11;1. He was having difficulty keeping up with his Grade 6 peers and, as documented by his teachers, had become disinterested in school work since undergoing tumour surgery. According to Phillip's mother, he had poor self-esteem and a limited concentration span.

TOLD-I

Phillip performed within normal limits on the TOLD-I despite the observation that he required particularly lengthy periods of time to respond to the test items.

Token Test for Children

Phillip scored within normal limits on all five parts of the *Token Test for Children*.

CELF

Phillip performed at age-appropriate levels for Subtests 7, 8 and 9 of the CELF.

BNT

A reduced naming ability was suggested by the BNT with Phillip's score of 35 falling below the normal range specified by the test.

TLC

Phillip performed below average on the high-level language tasks included in the TLC. He was unable to interpret and manipulate language at the level required in order to understand ambiguous sentences, make inferences, or recreate sentences. His understanding of metaphoric expressions was only just within normal limits.

Summary of language abilities

High-level language and naming deficits were demonstrated by Phillip.

Although he underwent two posterior fossa craniotomies, Phillip experienced no associated complications or CNS prophylaxis.

Case 11 (Brian)

Brian underwent the partial removal of an ependymoma at the age of 2;1. The tumour measured 3.4 cm in diameter, and was situated in the vermis passing towards the left side and downwards into the brainstem (see Figure 5.3). A VP shunt was also inserted at this time to alleviate obstructive hydrocephalus. Surgery was followed by courses of radiotherapy and chemotherapy. Chemotherapy involved eight cycles of CCNu (Iomustine) (40 mg on day 1), procarbazine (50 mg daily on days 8–21), and vincristine (7 mg on days 8–29). At the conclusion of treatment, there was no evidence of residual tumour on CT and Brian was described as cured.

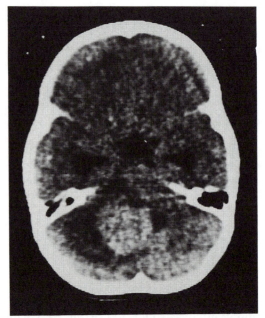

Figure 5.3 Case 11 (Brian): Pre-operative CT scan showing a posterior fossa ependymoma situated in the vermis and passing towards the left side. It measured 3.4 cm in diameter.

At the time of language assessment, Brian had been well for nine years two months since tumour removal and presented as a friendly co-operative 11-year-old child who was coping, but not excelling, in a normal Grade 5 class.

TOLD-I

Brian scored within the average range on all aspects of the TOLD-I. Although within normal limits, a reduction in language performance was documented by the Speaking and Syntax Quotients relative to the Quotients obtained for Listening and Semantics. This was due to the difficulty Brian experienced on the Sentence Combining and Word Ordering subtests.

Token Test for Children

With the exception of Part IV, Brian performed within normal limits on the *Token Test for Children*.

CELF

Brian performed above criteria on Subtests 7, 8 and 9 of the CELF.

BNT

Brian completed the BNT with ease, correctly naming 47 of the 60 items.

TLC

The TLC was attempted but abandoned due to the extreme difficulty Brian had in understanding the requirements of each subtest.

Summary of language abilities

Brian was the only subject included in the study reported by Murdoch and Hudson-Tennent (1994) who received both radiotherapy and chemotherapy following tumour resection. The administration of these two treatments in combination has been reported to contribute to language deficits (Norell et al., 1974; Kramer et al., 1988), and intellectual and learning disabilities (Holmes and Holmes, 1975; Meadows et al., 1981; Duffner et al., 1983). Brian, however, demonstrated relatively intact language skills nine years after tumour treatment.

Case 12 (William)

At the age of 9;9, William underwent the investigation of a 2-week history of vomiting and weight loss. A CT scan indicated the presence of a large, midline posterior fossa mass invading the vermis and fourth ventricle (see Figure 5.4). Complete surgical removal of a benign, cystic germinoma was performed. A right external ventricular drain remained in place for 4 days following surgery. William made a rapid, uneventful recovery and was discharged from hospital 10 days post-surgery. One week later, William was re-admitted to hospital due to the development of communicating hydrocephalus. This was relieved by lumbar puncture. No further complications or treatments were experienced.

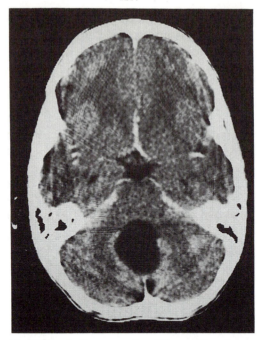

Figure 5.4 Case 12 (William): Pre-operative CT scan showing a midline posterior fossa germinoma invading the vermis and fourth ventricle.

William's language abilities were assessed at one year eight months after tumour removal. At that time he was healthy, had no evidence of residual or recurrent tumour, and at the age of 11;4, was successfully completing Grade 6 in a normal classroom situation.

TOLD-I

William performed within normal limits on all but one of the TOLD-I measures. Low average and below average scores on the Sentence Combining and Word Ordering Subtests, respectively, resulted in a Syntax Quotient of 83 being obtained.

Token Test for Children

No difficulty was experienced on the *Token Test for Children*, suggesting that impaired memory or attention did not contribute to the difficulties recorded on the TOLD-I subtests.

CELF

William performed above criterion on Subtests 7, 8 and 9 of the CELF.

BNT

The BNT normative data does not provide mean scores for children beyond the fifth grade. William who scored 48 correct performed at the upper end of the Grade 5 range of normal (37–48).

TLC

William scored within normal limits on all four subtests of the TLC.

Summary of language abilities

William did not require a VP shunt or CNS prophylaxis, but did experience recurrent hydrocephalus requiring hospital re-admission and lumbar puncture. Tasks that evaluated expressive syntax were most difficult for William, however, overall he demonstrated a competent level of language usage.

Case 13 (Anthony)

A 6-week history of intermittent frontal headaches, vomiting, ataxia and weight loss was experienced by Anthony prior to the diagnosis of a posterior fossa tumour. Anthony was aged 11;3 when a 4-cm mass involving the cerebellar vermis and fourth ventricle was detected by CT. Associated hydrocephalus was immediately treated by the surgical insertion of a right VP shunt. Three days later, a medulloblastoma was completely resected. Three days after tumour removal, Anthony became increasingly drowsy and irritable, and his speech deteriorated until he was unintelligible. A repeat CT scan failed to explain Anthony's condition, hence he was treated symptomatically with subsequent improvement. Anthony was discharged from hospital 10 weeks post-surgery following a course of craniospinal irradiation. He then attended a paediatric rehabilitation centre for 12 months where educational, speech therapy, occupational therapy and physiotherapy services were provided.

Language evaluation was performed two years one month post-surgery when Anthony was aged 13;4. He had returned to a regular primary school where, academically, he was coping in Grade 7. Remedial assistance was being provided for mathematics and library work.

TOLD-I and TOAL-2

Although the TOAL-2 was appropriate for Anthony's age, he was unable to complete this lengthy test. The five subtests he did complete allowed the calculation of three language quotients. Anthony obtained a Listening Quotient of 67, a Speaking Quotient of 82 and a Spoken Language Quotient of 72. All three quotients are below average. In particular, auditory comprehension skills fell below Anthony's expressive language abilities.

Anthony was able to complete the TOLD-I despite the heavy reliance on auditory skills imposed by this test. All quotients obtained on the TOLD-I were below the test's mean of 100 but were within the average range of 85–115. Again, Anthony's receptive language abilities were found to be poorer than his expressive skills.

Token Test for Children

Although the normative data provided by the *Token Test for Children* caters for children aged up to 12;6, this test was administered to Anthony due to his reduced comprehension scores on the TOLD series. His performance, as determined by the 12;6 norms, was within normal limits.

CELF

Subtests 7 and 9 were scored above criterion according to the test's normative data. The time pressure imposed on Subtest 8 resulted in Anthony making many errors and self-corrections when attempting to rapidly name the colours and shapes.

BNT

Anthony performed within normal limits on the BNT scoring 42 out of 60.

TLC

Anthony exhibited impairments of high-level language skills. All four subtests of the TLC were below average, and the overall standard score fell greater than 2 SD below the mean.

Summary of language abilities

Although Anthony performed within normal limits on most of the language tests, the administration of complex and high-level language tasks revealed impaired language competencies. Overall, Anthony's expressive language skills were in advance of his receptive abilities.

Case 14 (Nerida)

An extended symptom duration of approximately 12 months preceded Nerida's diagnosis of cerebellar medulloblastoma. Symptoms included headaches, dizziness, vomiting, personality changes, drowsiness, visual abnormalities, postural changes and reductions in school performance. At the age of 10;6, Nerida underwent the insertion of a right VP shunt followed by the total excision of a midline posterior fossa medulloblastoma. Surgical intervention resulted in a left lower motor neurone (VII) facial palsy, left divergent strabismus, and left hemiparesis. Following discharge from hospital 1 month post-surgery Nerida was administered a 6-week course of craniospinal irradiation involving a total dose of 5000 rads delivered in 28 fractions. At the conclusion of treatment, Nerida was enrolled in a paediatric rehabilitation centre where she received daily speech therapy, physiotherapy, occupational therapy and special education services for a period of 8 months.

At the time of language testing, at age 12;10, Nerida had repeated Grade 6, and had been placed in a normal Grade 7 class where she was experiencing severe academic and social difficulties. She exhibited residual ataxia, hemiplegia, facial palsy and strabismus.

TOLD-I and TOAL-2

Both the TOLD-I and TOAL-2 were administered due to Nerida's age. The results indicated that while Nerida scored below average on both language tests, she experienced greater difficulty with the more advanced language tasks included in the TOAL-2.

Token Test for Children

Despite exceeding the age limit on the *Token Test for Children* by four months, Nerida's performance on the TOLD series indicated a need to administer this test, rather than the *Token Test*, which is usually used for older subjects. According to the age 12;6 norms, Nerida scored below average on the *Token Test for Children*. All of Nerida's errors involved confusing the colour and/or shape of the token to be manipulated with another token described in the same command or in a previous command. Nerida did not confuse any of the concepts tested in Part V.

CELF

Nerida was successfully able to complete the rapid language retrieval and production tasks of the CELF.

BNT

Nerida scored within normal limits on the BNT, correctly naming 44 of the 60 items.

TLC

Although Nerida was able to identify the two meanings of an ambiguous sentence, she was unable to infer or interpret information that was not specifically provided (i.e. Subtests 2 and 4), nor was she able to generate sentences when given three stimulus words and a situation.

Summary of language abilities

Nerida evidenced a global language deficit, which became increasingly apparent as more difficult language tasks were attempted.

Case 15 (Warren)

At the age of 10;10, Warren underwent neurological assessments to investigate a 3-week history of poor concentration, 6 days of frequent headaches, and 3 days of vomiting, clumsiness and diplopia. A large midline mass in the inferior vermis associated with a moderate degree of hydrocephalus was revealed by CT. An ependymoma was partially excised and an external ventricular drain inserted. A VP shunt was not required. Warren made a slow but steady recovery. Surgery was followed by a course of craniospinal irradiation involving a total dose of 5000 rads administered in 30 fractions. A CT scan obtained 2 months post-irradiation showed normal ventricular size and an absence of residual tumour.

At the time of assessment two years three months post-surgery, Warren was free of recurrent tumour and exhibited only a mild residual gait ataxia. His most recent Grade 8 examination results included an A+ for Science, Mathematics and Manual Arts and a B+ for English, Geography and Home Economics.

TOAL-2

All language quotients obtained on the TOAL-2 were within normal limits.

CELF

Performances on all three subtests of the CELF were above criterion.

BNT

Warren was unable to name only three of the 60 BNT items. All three items were named after a phonemic cue was provided by the examiner.

TLC

Warren demonstrated an average performance on the TLC. Making inferences from a limited amount of given information was the most difficult task for Warren while identifying the alternative meanings of ambiguous sentences presented few difficulties.

Summary of language abilities

Despite a history of hydrocephalus, tumour, surgery, CNS irradiation, and a reportedly slow recovery, Warren demonstrated an age-appropriate level of language competence and a high standard of academic achievement. Several studies have determined a lower risk of long-term deficits in children treated for tumour when older than 10 years (Bamford et al., 1976; Danoff et al., 1982; Packer et al., 1989; Hoppe-Hirsch et al., 1990). Warren's age at diagnosis may have been a favourable prognostic factor in this case. In addition, an early diagnosis as indicated by the reportedly short pre-morbid history of three weeks may have limited the effects of hydrocephalus and tumour size.

Case 16 (Julie)

Julie, a female aged 6;8, experienced a history of inco-ordination, papilloedema and vomiting prior to hospital admission and examination. A CT scan performed 1 day after admission revealed a large enhancing tumour in the midline of the posterior fossa extending up into the superior vermis (see Figure 5.5). It was slightly larger on the left than the right. A considerable amount of surrounding oedema was observed as well as compression of the fourth ventricle due to hydrocephalus. A posterior fossa craniotomy was then performed and complete tumour resection was possible. Final diagnosis was that of a solid cerebellar astrocytoma. Julie experienced an uneventful post-operative recovery. As a low grade astrocytoma was diagnosed radiotherapy was not required.

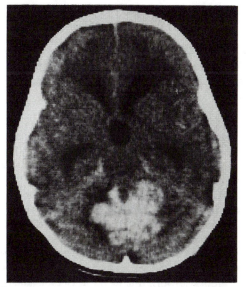

Figure 5.5 Case 16 (Julie): Pre-operative CT scan showing a large astrocytoma in the midline of the posterior fossa. It is slightly larger on the left than on the right.

At the time of language assessment, seven years three months post-surgery, Julie presented as an alert girl aged 13;11 who expressed enthusiasm towards school and her many extra-curricular activities. She had just completed Grade 9 and had received outstanding results for all subjects, except Mathematics for which an average score was achieved.

TOAL-2

An Overall Language Quotient of 107 was achieved on the TOAL-2 and all other language quotients were within the average range.

CELF

Performance on all three subtests of rapid language retrieval and production was within normal limits.

BNT

Julie spontaneously named all but three of the 60 BNT items. These items were retrieved immediately following the provision of a phonemic cue.

TLC

Julie obtained average scores on all four subtests of the TLC.

Summary of language abilities

Julie presented as a high achiever in the areas of sport, music and school performance. With respect to language, Julie performed within normal limits or above average on all of the language tests administered.

Case 17 (Marcus)

Following a 1-month history of unsteady gait and intermittent headaches, vomiting and blurring of vision, Marcus collapsed and hit his head. A CT scan identified a calcified tumour of the fourth ventricle and associated hydro-cephalus (see Figure 5.6). Marcus underwent surgery for the insertion of a right external ventricular drain and subtotal removal of a medulloblastoma. The tumour was found to fill the fourth ventricle, obstruct the aqueduct and was adherent to the right wall of the fourth ventricle. Marcus made a rapid recovery and was discharged from hospital 7 days post-surgery. A CT scan performed at the conclusion of craniospinal irradiation showed no evidence of residual ventricular tumour. Eight months post-treatment, a CT scan revealed mild cerebral atrophy due to whole brain irradiation but no signs of recurrent or residual tumour.

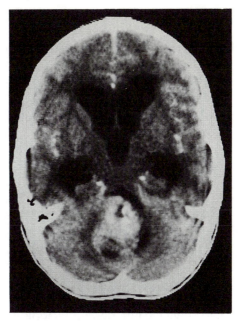

Figure 5.6 Case 17 (Marcus): Pre-operative CT scan showing a calcified medulloblastoma of the fourth ventricle and associated hydrocephalus.

Language assessment was carried out at one year eleven months post-surgery, at which time Marcus, aged 14;11, was experiencing moderate academic difficulties in a normal Grade 9 class.

TOAL-2

All but one of the language quotients obtained by Marcus fell greater than 2 SD below the test mean. His expressive semantic and syntactic skills were marginally above the other language measures as reflected by the Speaking Quotient. Examination of the specific TOAL-2 subtests indicated that most difficulty was experienced comprehending spoken and written syntactic structures, as well as writing grammatically correct sentences.

Token Test for Children

Although Marcus was aged 14;11 at the time of testing, the *Token Test for Children* was administered to supplement the information provided by the TOAL-2. His auditory comprehension abilities were shown to be below average relative to the data provided for children aged 12;6. Marcus made errors in token selection and in the concepts presented in Part V.

CELF

All three timed subtests of the CELF were scored above criteria.

BNT

Marcus performed within normal limits, correctly naming 41 of the 60 items on the BNT.

TLC

Overall, Marcus performed poorly on tasks involving high-level language competencies. A standard score within the normal range was obtained for Subtest 3 (Recreating Sentences), which corresponds to his best performance on the TOAL-2 — Subtest IV (Speaking/Grammar).

Summary of language abilities

The global reduction in language functioning, as indicated by the TOAL-2, the *Token Test for Children* and the TLC, could have been anticipated in the presence of the generalized cerebral atrophy revealed by CT. Receptive language skills were slightly more impaired than expressive abilities.

Case 18 (Ben)

Ben presented for neurological examination at the age of 13;3 following a 2-month history of headaches, slurred speech and mild ataxia. A CT scan showed an infiltrating, low density, mass lesion in the cerebellum (see Figure 5.7). Marked hydrocephalus was also present. A VP shunt was inserted to alleviate the hydrocephalus, and 1 week later an ependymoma was partially removed. Immediately following surgery, truncal ataxia was observed but speech was described as clear. Recovery was rapid and Ben was discharged 6 days after tumour excision. A course of craniospinal irradiation followed, involving a total radiation dose of 5000 rads. A CT scan performed at the conclusion of treatment indicated the presence of residual ependymoma in the superior vermian cistern and mild ventromegaly. No further treatment was provided.

At the time of his language assessment two years four months post-surgery, Ben was in Grade 10. Parental and school reports indicated that although Ben had been a very high achiever pre-morbidly, he was now failing all subjects.

TOAL-2

Most of the language quotients obtained by Ben were within the test's normal range. Listening/Grammar was the only subtest for which a below average standard score was obtained and as a result, a below

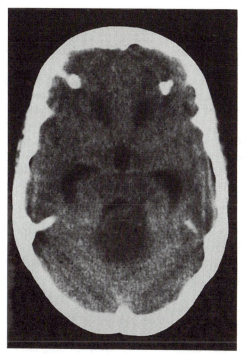

Figure 5.7 Case 18 (Ben): Pre-operative CT scan showing a posterior fossa ependymoma in the midline and slightly to the left of the midline.

average auditory comprehension (Listening) Quotient was recorded as well as low-average Receptive Language (auditory and reading comprehension) and Grammar Quotients.

CELF

All three tests of rapid language retrieval and production were scored above criteria.

BNT

Ben correctly named 56 of the 60 BNT items.

TLC

Ben demonstrated an average level of language competency as determined by the TLC.

Summary of language abilities

Ben made a rapid recovery following partial resection of an ependymoma. Overall, he exhibited intact language skills.

Case 19 (Brett)

Brett underwent total excision of a cystic astrocytoma (Grade III) of the cerebellar vermis when he was aged 12;3. Tumour diagnosis was preceded by a 4-week history of nausea, vomiting, fainting and intermittent headaches. Neurological examination revealed a mild right upper motor neurone VII nerve paresis with resultant left facial weakness and reduced movement of the right side of the soft palate. Speech was described as normal. Post-operatively, Brett responded slowly due to persistent vomiting and subsequent dehydration. Fifteen days post-surgery, Brett commenced a course of craniospinal irradiation involving a total dose of 5000 rads delivered in 28 fractions over 42 days. As Brett lived in a country town, he underwent radiotherapy as an in-patient, and was discharged from hospital eight and a half weeks after tumour diagnosis.

At the time of his language assessment, three years ten months post-surgery, Brett was achieving above average grades for all Grade 11 subjects. He had been elected school captain for his senior year and had ambitions to study either Accountancy or English at University.

TOAL-2

Brett achieved average or above average quotients on all components of the TOAL-2.

CELF

Subtests 7, 8 and 9 of the CELF subtests were scored above criteria.

BNT

Brett correctly named 54 of the 60 items of the BNT, which was within the normative range.

Summary of language abilities

Brett demonstrated a high level of competency in all aspects of language assessed despite experiencing a high grade tumour, neurosurgery and CNS irradiation. Two factors that may have contributed to Brett's favourable prognosis include the older age (12;3) at which he was diagnosed and treated and the fact that the hydrocephalus that he experienced did not require the insertion of a shunt as treatment.

Case 20 (Peter)

Peter experienced a 6-month history of vomiting, headaches and coughing, followed by the development of ataxia, prior to the diagnosis of a cerebellar juvenile astrocytoma at age 12;1. Following surgery to insert a right VP shunt, Peter was drowsy and exhibited a left facial paresis and left upper limb paresis. No improvement occurred before the posterior fossa craniotomy was performed 13 days later. An astrocytoma, 5 cm in diameter, was completely resected from the midline and left side of the cerebellum. Peter was mute post-surgery and exhibited a poor recovery. Three days after tumour removal, he became cyanosed due to a collapsed left lung and had to be re-intubated for 2 days. One week after this incident, Peter was still drowsy and exhibited a left hemiparesis but was able to move all limbs on request. A CT scan revealed a right-sided extradural haemorrhage which was immediately evacuated with resultant improved consciousness. One month after tumour removal, a follow-up CT scan revealed the presence of a densely calcified membrane associated with a right-sided epidural collection. The collection did not appear to have as much mass effect as the previous extradural haemorrhage. The collection and calcified membrane were removed at a fourth operation. Peter exhibited a more rapid recovery than was previously experienced. His hemiparesis resolved, however, he remained ataxic. At this time, he was able to obey simple commands and identify some body parts. Two shunt revisions were required during the 4 years following tumour removal. Three years after the initial surgery, recurrent astrocytoma was detected adjacent to the left cerebellar peduncle. This was subtotally resected, after which a rapid, uneventful recovery was made. Neither radiotherapy nor chemotherapy were included in Peter's treatment regimen.

At the time of language assessment, four years nine months after tumour diagnosis, Peter evidenced a small residual tumour in the posterior fossa, which was being regularly monitored. He was ataxic and used a wheelchair most of the time. His co-ordination and hearing were deteriorating as the need for further surgery approached. Peter had withdrawn from school at the age of 15. According to his parents, Peter had been an excellent scholar prior to tumour diagnosis.

TOAL-2

Due to poor vision and a marked fine motor deficit, Peter was unable to complete the five subtests of the TOAL-2 which involved reading, writing and picture stimuli. Subtests II (Listening/Grammar), III (Speaking/Vocabulary) and IV (Speaking/Grammar) were completed, resulting in a Speaking Quotient of 82. No other language quotients could be calculated. Peter's comprehension of syntax (Subtest III) was shown to be in advance of his expressive syntactic abilities (Subtest IV).

CELF

Although Subtest 7 was scored above criterion, Subtests 8 and 9 were scored below criterion on the CELF. The presence of a severe dysarthria inhibited the rapid production of language during these tasks.

BNT

Impaired vision prevented Peter's completion of the BNT.

TLC

Fatigue and an inability to see the written and picture stimuli included in the TLC prevented the administration of this test.

Summary of language abilities

Peter presented with severe communication and physical disabilities. The TOAL-2 indicated the presence of an expressive language deficit, which may have been exacerbated by Peter's attempts to overcome poor intelligibility. Factors that may have contributed to Peter's poor functional status include the additional surgical procedures experienced, the episode of cyanosis, the mass effect of the extradural haemorrhage and the epidural collection, the recurrent tumour and the prolonged pre-morbid symptoms which were most likely signs of hydrocephalus.

It is noteworthy that Peter exhibited severe language problems despite the presence of several factors in his history that would normally imply a good prognosis. These factors include, his relatively older age at diagnosis, tumour type and lack of chemotherapy and radiotherapy in his treatment regimen.

Nature and severity of language impairment following treatment for posterior fossa tumours in children

An examination of 20 tumour cases outlined above demonstrates very clearly that the nature and severity of language impairment following treatment for a posterior fossa tumour in childhood varies widely from case to case. Only three subjects (Cases 8, 14 and 17) exhibited a global language deficit as indicated by a uniform reduction across all receptive and expressive language skills. Five of the children (Cases 4, 9, 15, 16 and 19) demonstrated a competent standard of language usage. The remaining 12 children were shown to have strengths and weaknesses across the various language abilities that were assessed.

Six of the children treated for tumours (Cases 3, 5, 7, 11, 12 and 20) exhibited particular difficulties with expressive semantic and/or syntactic language tasks. A reduction in expressive language abilities has been identified by several authors as a characteristic of acquired aphasia in children resulting from various aetiologies, including tumour (Alajouanine and Lhermitte, 1965; Satz and Bullard-Bates, 1981;

Carrow-Woolfolk and Lynch, 1982; Van Dongen et al., 1985; Cooper and Flowers, 1987; Jordan et al., 1988). A common expressive deficit identified in children with acquired CNS aetiologies is poor word-finding ability (Carrow-Woolfolk and Lynch, 1982; Hécaen, 1983; Visch-Brink and van de Sandt-Koenderman, 1984; Cooper and Flowers, 1987; Martins and Ferro, 1987; Van Dongen and Visch-Brink, 1988; Jordan et al., 1990). Hudson and Murdoch (1992) previously reported that, when considered as a group, the naming abilities of the 20 tumour subjects were not significantly below those of a group of age- and sex-matched control subjects. When considered individually, however, seven of the tumour subjects did perform poorly on the CELF subtests and/or the BNT (Cases 2, 5, 6, 7, 8, 10 and 13). Difficulties encountered included an extended period of time required to complete the task, as well as an inability to access the correct names of items that were either requested or pictured.

Five subjects exhibited language deficits that were predominantly receptive in nature (Cases 1, 2, 6, 13 and 18). Several authors have reported comprehension difficulties in acquired childhood aphasia to be either relatively uncommon or likely to resolve in the long term (Alajouanine and Lhermitte, 1965; Pohl, 1979; Carrow-Woolfolk and Lynch, 1982; Aram et al., 1983; Hécaen, 1983; Van Dongen et al., 1985). More recent studies, however, have systematically examined receptive skills using batteries of standardized tests and have identified long-term deficits in children suffering various acquired aetiologies (Visch-Brink and van de Sandt-Koenderman, 1984; Van Hout and Lyon, 1986; Cooper and Flowers, 1987). Based on the 20 cases described above, it is suggested that, in children treated for posterior fossa tumour, long-term comprehension difficulties are just as likely to occur as long-term expressive deficits.

Factors influencing language outcomes in children treated for posterior fossa tumours

The performance of each of the tumour subjects outlined above on the language tests may have been influenced by a number of variables relating to their medical condition and treatment. In particular, factors such as the inclusion of CNS prophylaxis in their treatment protocols, their age at diagnosis, the type of tumour experienced, the occurrence of associated hydrocephalus and the duration of pre-surgical symptoms (e.g. headache, vomiting, diplopia and nystagmus) may have affected their language scores. The administration of CNS prophylaxis has been reported to affect the long-term functional abilities of paediatric cancer patients (Meadows et al., 1981; Danoff et al., 1982; Copeland et al., 1985; Duffner et al., 1985). Radiation-induced damage has reportedly developed in children irradiated for CNS tumours up to 14 years after the completion of treatment (Lee and Suh, 1977) and has included cerebral atrophy, calcification, necrosis and cerebrovascular damage. Three subjects described above (Cases 3, 7 and 17) demonstrated CT evidence of structural damage to the brain attributable to radiotherapy. A fourth subject (Case 18) was diagnosed with long-standing periventricular demyelination 14 months after his involvement in the study. It is possible that this condition may have been present during the language assessment procedures. All four subjects with proven radiation-induced cerebral damage exhibited language difficulties, which may have resulted from such damage.

Although the language status of the four children who had suffered radiation-induced CNS damage supports the hypothesis that language impairments occur subsequent to craniospinal radiotherapy, consideration of the remaining 16 subjects does not provide such conclusive evidence. Cases 6, 10, 12 and 20 did not undergo craniospinal irradiation and yet did exhibit varying degrees of language impairment. For example, Case 10 demonstrated a word-finding deficit and difficulties with high-level language tasks, whereas Case 6 exhibited reduced language scores in most areas tested with particular difficulties being experienced during tasks of receptive semantics and syntax. The remaining two subjects who did not undergo a course of radiotherapy (Cases 4 and 16) demonstrated intact language skills across all measures.

Consideration of the subjects who did experience craniospinal irradiation also fails to provide conclusive support for a radiation related explanation of language impairments. For example, Cases 9, 15 and 19 each received a total radiation dose of 5000 rads to the brain and spinal cord and yet achieved age-appropriate scores on all language measures. The results of the study described above, therefore, suggest that the presence of CNS radiotherapy in the treatment protocol is not necessarily indicative of a negative prognosis for long-term language skills.

The long-term functional abilities of children given CNS prophylaxis may also be related to the age at which radiotherapy was administered. Several researchers have suggested that the younger the child is at the time of CNS irradiation, the greater the risk of long-term structural and functional CNS damage (Danoff et al., 1982; Pearson et al., 1983; Davis et al., 1986; Packer et al., 1989; Hoppe-Hirsch et al., 1990). For instance, studies of intellectual functioning have suggested that children with tumours who are less than six years of age at diagnosis and treatment have a greater risk of intellectual deterioration than those older than six years (Danoff et al., 1982; Mulhern and Kun, 1985). The same may be true of language abilities. In support of this suggestion, six of the seven tumour children reported above who were less than five years of age when treated with CNS irradiation exhibited language problems (Cases 1, 2, 3, 6, 7 and 8). However, five of the children older than five years at the time of treatment also exhibited chronic language deficits, including four children who were older than 10 years when administered radiotherapy.

The failure of CNS irradiation to fully explain the varied language performances of the tumour group suggests that factors other than radiotherapy must also have influenced the language status of the tumour cases. All 20 subjects described by Murdoch and Hudson-Tennent (1994) experienced hydrocephalus prior to tumour diagnosis. Language deficits subsequent to increased intracranial pressure have been reported, particularly in children suffering neural tube disorders (Dennis et al., 1987; Henderson et al., 1989). Various receptive and expressive language characteristics have been described in studies of children suffering hydrocephalus, however, a common observation across studies has been the lack of uniformity in the level of ability demonstrated by subjects across different aspects of language functioning (Tew et al., 1979; Billard et al., 1986; Dennis et al., 1987; Henderson et al., 1989). It has been found that children with hydrocephalus may exhibit a particular weakness in either their receptive or expressive language skills. The majority of the 20 subjects treated for posterior fossa tumours described above also exhibited specific language strengths and weaknesses, rather than a uniform reduction in all language skills.

Another factor that might have influenced the language abilities of the 20 tumour children is the duration of hydrocephalus. The longest symptom duration (one year) was experienced by Case 14 who also demonstrated a severe language disturbance (most language scores fell greater than 2 SD below the mean). Case 20 experienced hydrocephalic symptoms for 24 weeks before tumour diagnosis and was found to have below average expressive language abilities. Case 20 did, however, experience several other complications (such as cyanosis) that may account for his disabilities. Others who experienced prolonged symptom durations included Case 8 (12 weeks) and Case 10 (10 weeks). Case 8 demonstrated the most severely disordered language skills of all 20 subjects assessed, whereas Case 10 exhibited only word-finding deficits and impaired performance on advanced language tasks. The remaining 16 subjects were reported to have symptom durations lasting between two and eight weeks. Overall, therefore, the results tend to suggest that prolonged periods of hydrocephalus may have detrimental effects on long-term language abilities.

The treatment of hydrocephalus using shunts has also been reported to affect children's language abilities (Dennis et al., 1987; Query et al., 1990). Dennis et al. (1987) determined shunt treatment to be a predictor of poor word fluency and automaticity in their group of 75 children and adolescents who had experienced hydrocephalus during the first year of life. Query et al. (1990) interviewed 36 adolescents who had received shunts to alleviate hydrocephalus when less than two years of age and reported poor comprehension, word-finding deficits and the need for academic assistance and/or speech/language intervention. Only three subjects reported by Murdoch and Hudson-Tennent (1994) did not undergo shunt insertion for the treatment of hydrocephalus (Cases 10, 17 and 19). These three subjects represent a full range of language abilities from severely language disordered (Case 17), to mildly impaired (Case 10) to above average skills (Case 19). Hence the influence of shunt insertion is difficult to ascertain.

The long-term quality of life experienced by children treated for posterior fossa tumour is considered to be more favourable for those children diagnosed with either cystic or juvenile astrocytomas (Gjerris and Klinken, 1978; Wallner et al., 1988) and for those children who undergo total excision of the tumour (regardless of its type) (Gol, 1963; Laws et al., 1987; Wallner et al., 1988; Garcia et al., 1990). Based on these findings, it may be anticipated that Cases 4, 10, 16, 19 and 20 would function without any serious disability. Certainly, cases 4, 16 and 19 demonstrated exceptional language, academic and social skills. Case 10 exhibited only high-level language deficits but was experiencing academic difficulties. Case 20, however, required full-time care and, based on a limited assessment, was considered to have an expressive language deficit. Case 20 did, however, experience several complications following tumour excision (e.g. extradural haemorrhages, shunt failure, cyanosis and residual tumour) which no doubt contributed to his disabilities. Of the remaining 15 tumour children, only Case 9 and Case 15 demonstrated intact language skills. Case 9 had experienced the partial removal of a medulloblastoma, whereas Case 15 had had an ependymoma partially excised. Thus, the total surgical excision of an astrocytoma may suggest a favourable language prognosis in the long term, however, children with other tumour types and different extents of surgery also have the potential to maintain competent levels of language usage in the long term.

It is apparent from the reported case studies that the many complex factors associated with the presence and management of posterior fossa tumours cannot, in isolation, account for the language deficits that were identified in the group of tumour patients described in the present chapter. Each of these factors can be considered to contribute to the overall outcome of posterior fossa tumour treatment. The results of the 20 cases reported by Murdoch and Hudson-Tennent (1994) indicate that the language skills of all children who experience tumour treatment should be monitored in the long term and the appropriate intervention provided.

References

Alajouanine T, Lhermitte F (1965) Acquired aphasia in children. Brain 88: 653–662.
Aram DM, Rose DF, Rekate HL, Whitaker HA (1983) Acquired capsular/striatal aphasias in childhood. Archives of Neurology 40: 614–617.

Bamford FN, Morris-Jones P, Pearson D, Ribeiro GG, Shalet SM, Beardwell CG (1976) Residual disabilities in children treated for intracranial space-occupying lesions. Cancer 37: 1149–1151.

Billard C, Santini JJ, Gillet P, Nargeot MC, Adrien JC (1986) Long term intellectual prognosis of hydrocephalus with reference to 77 children. Pediatric Neuroscience 12: 219–225.

Carrow-Woolfolk E, Lynch J (1982) An Integrated Approach to Language Disorders in Children. Orlando, FL: Grune & Stratton.

Cooper JA, Flowers CR (1987) Children with a history of acquired aphasia: residual language and academic impairments. Journal of Speech and Hearing Disorders 52: 251–262.

Copeland DR, Fletcher JM, Pfefferbaum-Levine B, Jaffe N, Reid H, Maor N (1985) Neuropsychological sequelae of childhood cancer in long-term survivors. Pediatrics 75: 745–753.

Danoff BF, Chowchock FS, Marquette C, Mulgrew L, Kramer S (1982) Assessment of the long-term effects of primary radiation therapy for brain tumours in children. Cancer 49: 1580–1586.

Davis PC, Hoffman JC, Pearl GS, Braun IF (1986) CT evaluation of effects of cranial radiation therapy in children. American Journal of Roentgenology 147: 587–592.

Dennis ME, Hendricks B, Hoffman HJ, Humphreys RP (1987) Language of hydrocephalic children and adolescents. Journal of Clinical and Experimental Neuropsychology 9: 593–621.

DiSimoni F (1978) The Token Test for Children. Hingham, MA: Teaching Resources.

Duffner PK, Cohen ME, Thomas PRM (1983) Late effects of treatment on the intelligence of children with posterior fossa tumours. Cancer 51: 233–237.

Duffner PK, Cohen ME, Thomas RM, Lansky SB (1985) The long-term effects of cranial irradiation on the central nervous system. Cancer 56: 1841–1846.

Garcia DM, Marks JE, Latifi HR, Klieforth B (1990) Childhood cerebellar astrocytomas: is there a role for postoperative irradiation? International Journal of Radiation Oncology Biology Physics 18: 815—818.

Gjerris F, Klinken L (1978) Long-term prognosis in children with benign cerebellar astrocytoma. Journal of Neurosurgery 49: 179–184.

Gol A (1963) Cerebellar astrocytomas in children. American Journal of Diseases of Childhood 106: 21–24.

Hammill DD, Newcomer PL (1982) Test of Language Development — Intermediate. Austin, TX: Pro-Ed.

Hammill DD, Brown VL, Larsen SC, Wiederhold JL (1987) Test of Adolescent Language 2: A Multidimensional Approach to Assessment. Austin, TX: Pro-Ed.

Hécaen H (1983) Acquired aphasia in children: revisited. Neuropsychologia 21: 581–587.

Henderson S, Murdoch BE, Ozanne AE (1989) Speech and language disorders in children with spina bifida. Paper presented at the Annual Conference of the Australian Association of Speech and Hearing, Perth.

Hodges S, Smithells RW (1983) Intercranial calcification and childhood medulloblastoma. Archives of Disease in Childhood 58: 663–664.

Holmes HA, Holmes FF (1975) After ten years, what are the handicaps and lifestyles of children treated for cancer? An examination of the present status of 124 survivors. Clinical Pediatrics 14: 819–823.

Hoppe-Hirsch E, Renier D, Lellouch-Tubiana A, Sainte-Rose C, Pierre-Kahn A, Hirsch JF (1990) Medulloblastoma in childhood: progressive intellectual deterioration. Child's Nervous System 6: 60–65.

Hudson LJ, Murdoch BE (1992) Chronic language deficits in children treated for posterior fossa tumours. Aphasiology 6: 135–150.

Jordan FM, Ozanne AE, Murdoch BE (1988) Long term speech and language disorders subsequent to closed head injury in children. Brain Injury 2: 179–185.

Jordan FM, Ozanne AE, Murdoch BE (1990) Performance of closed head-injured children on a naming task. Brain Injury 4: 27–32.

Kaplan E, Goodglass H, Weintraub S (1983) Boston Naming Test. Philadelphia, PA: Lea & Febiger.

Kramer JH, Norman D, Brant-Zawadski M, Ablin A, Moore IM (1988) Absence of white matter changes on magnetic resonance imaging in children treated with CNS prophylaxis therapy for leukaemia. Cancer 61: 928–930.

Laws ER, Bergstralh EJ, Taylor WF (1987) Cerebellar astrocytoma in children. Progress in Experimental Tumour Research 30: 122–127.

Lee KF, Suh JH (1977) CT evidence of grey matter calcification secondary to radiation therapy. Computerized Tomography 1: 103–110.

Martins IP, Ferro JM (1987) Acquired conduction aphasia in a child. Developmental Medicine and Child Neurology 29: 529–540.

Meadows AT, Massari DJ, Ferguson J, Gordon J, Littman P, Moss K (1981) Declines in IQ scores and cognitive dysfunctions in children with acute lymphocytic leukaemia treated with cranial irradiation. Lancet ii: 1015–1018.

Mulhern RK, Kun LE (1985) Neuropsychologic function in children with brain tumours. III. Interval changes in the six months following treatment. Medical and Pediatric Oncology 13: 318–324.

Murdoch BE, Hudson-Tennent LJ (1994) Differential language outcomes in children following treatment for posterior fossa tumours. Aphasiology 8: 507–534.

Newcomer PL, Hammill DD (1982) Test of Language Development — Primary. Austin, TX: Pro-Ed.

Norrell H, Wilson CB, Slagel DE, Clark DB (1974) Leukoencephalopathy following the administration of methotrexate into the cerebrospinal fluid in the treatment of primary brain tumours. Cancer 33: 923–932.

Packer RJ, Sutton LN, Atkins TE, Radcliffe J, Bunin GR, D'Angio G, Siegel KR, Schut L (1989) A prospective study of cognitive function in children receiving whole-brain radiotherapy and chemotherapy: 2-year results. Journal of Neurosurgery 70: 707–713.

Pearson ADJ, Campbell AN, McAllister VL, Pearson GL (1983) Intracranial calcification in survivors of childhood medulloblastoma. Archives of Disease in Childhood 58: 133–136.

Pohl P (1979) Dichotic listening in a child recovering from acquired aphasia. Brain and Language 8: 372–379.

Query JM, Reichelt C, Christopherson LA (1990) Living with chronic illness: a retrospective study of patients shunted for hydrocephalus and their families. Developmental Medicine and Child Neurology 32: 119–128.

Satz P, Bullard-Bates C (1981) Acquired aphasia in children. In Sarno MT (ed.) Acquired Aphasia. New York: Academic Press: 398–426.

Semel EM, Wiig EH (1982) Clinical Evaluation of Language Functions. Columbus, OH: Charles E Merrill.

Tew B (1979). The 'cocktail party syndrome' in children with hydrocephalus and spina bifida. British Journal of Disorders of Communication 14: 89–101.

Van Dongen HR, Visch-Brink EG (1988) Naming in aphasic children: analysis of paraphasic errors. Neuropsychologia 26: 629–632.

Van Dongen HR, Loonen CB, Van Dongen KJ (1985) Anatomical basis for acquired fluent aphasia in children. Annals of Neurology 17: 306–309.

Van Hout A, Lyon G (1986) Wernicke's aphasia in a 10 year old boy. Brain and Language 29: 268–285.

Visch-Brink EG, van de Sandt-Koenderman M (1984) The occurrence of paraphasias in the spontaneous speech of children with acquired aphasia. Brain and Language 23: 256–271.

Wallner KE, Gonzales MF, Edwards MS, Wara WM, Sheline GE (1988) Treatment results of juvenile pilocytic astrocytoma. Journal of Neurosurgery 69: 171–176.

Wiig EH, Secord W (1985) Test of Language Competence. Columbus, OH: Charles E Merrill.

Chapter 6
Language disorders in children treated for acute lymphoblastic leukaemia

BRUCE E MURDOCH AND DEBORAH L BOON

Introduction

Treatment of acute lymphoblastic leukaemia (ALL) is aimed at inducing, consolidating and maintaining remission of the disease, and involves multi-drug chemotherapy and sometimes radiotherapy. As discussed in Chapter 2, this treatment is often followed by a number of adverse sequelae, many of which have the potential to disrupt normal language function. Among these adverse sequelae are both structural and functional changes in the brain.

Studies using computerized tomography (CT) have identified a number of structural brain abnormalities in leukaemic patients who have received central nervous system (CNS) prophylaxis. These abnormalities, which are grouped together as leucoencephalopathy (disease of the white matter of the brain), include: hypodensity of white matter attributed to demyelination; ventricular dilation; and cerebral calcifications (Peylan-Ramu et al., 1978; Pizzo et al., 1979; Ochs et al., 1980, 1986). Microangiopathies (calcification of cerebral blood vessels) have also been identified in patients treated with cranial radiation (2400 rads), and intrathecal (IT) and intravenous methotrexate (MTX) (Price and Birdwell, 1978; Ch'ien et al., 1981).

In addition to causing structural abnormalities, CNS prophylaxis may also have detrimental effects on various neuropsychological functions. Several investigators have described intellectual impairment in children treated for ALL with cranial irradiation and chemotherapy (Eiser, 1978; Meadows et al., 1981; Duffner et al., 1985; Said et al., 1987; Taylor et al., 1987). Duffner et al. (1983) and Taylor et al. (1987) noted a subtle but significant lowering of intelligence quotients (IQs) in long-term survivors of ALL. CNS prophylaxis, in the form of cranial irradiation or the combination of radiotherapy and IT MTX, is a primary factor in the development of the reported mild neuropsychological deficits (Eiser, 1978; Tamaroff et al., 1982; Tebbi, 1982).

Twaddle et al. (1983) estimated pre-treatment intelligence quotients (IQs) of leukaemic and solid tumour patients treated with a combination of MTX and cranial radiation (2400 rads) from corrected measures of sibling IQ. A significant difference between these estimates and post-treatment IQs was found in the ALL group, but not in the solid tumour group. Twaddle et al. (1983) noted that aspects of intelligence, such as verbal associate reasoning and reasoning with abstract material, were particularly vulnerable.

Considering the disruption of intelligence noted by Twaddle et al. (1983), it is likely that subtle deficits in language function also occur in children treated for leukaemia. Unfortunately, most statements regarding the language abilities of children treated for ALL are based on neuropsychological measures rather than a comprehensive linguistic assessment. Consequently, although a number of authors have noted that language is spared by CNS prophylaxis in childhood leukaemia (Eiser, 1978, 1980; Brouwers et al., 1985; Copeland et al., 1985), effects on language may have been missed due to the lack of sufficiently sensitive or specifically designed measures of language. In support of this latter suggestion, Taylor et al. (1987) identified problems with language in children with acute lymphoblastic leukaemia post-irradiation. These researchers used four age-normed assessments of language (the *Expressive One Word Picture Vocabulary Test*, the *Token Test*, the *Word Fluency Test* and the *Verbal Selective Reminding Test*) and reported that leukaemic subjects performed less well than their siblings on tasks requiring speed and accuracy (word fluency, contingency naming) and on a task requiring an ability to follow multiple step direction (*Token Test*). Mild linguistic deficits were also reported to occur in nine children treated for ALL tested by Jackel et al. (1990) on a battery of tests sensitive to high-level language function. Consequently, although the findings of studies based on neuropsychological assessments have indicated that language is spared by CNS prophylaxis, the results of Jackel et al. (1990) and Taylor et al. (1987) indicate that linguistic deficits may be demonstrated in children treated for ALL when tested with appropriate measures of linguistic function.

To date, the most extensive investigations of the language abilities of children treated for ALL are those carried out by Buttsworth et al. (1993) and Murdoch et al. (1994). Specifically, Buttsworth et al. (1993) compared the performance of a group of 22 children treated for leukaemia on a battery of language tests with that of a group of age- and sex-matched non-neurologically impaired control subjects. Murdoch et al. (1994) documented the individual variability in language outcomes demonstrated by children treated for ALL through a detailed case-by-case examination of 23 such children.

The procedures used by Buttsworth et al. (1993) and Murdoch et al. (1994), together with the major findings of these two studies, are outlined below.

Language impairments following treatment for leukaemia: evidence from group studies

As a follow-up to the preliminary study reported by Jackel et al. (1990), Buttsworth et al. (1993) examined the language abilities of a larger group (N=22) of children treated for ALL. The subjects included ranged in age from 5;0 to 17;9, with a mean age of 11;2 (SD = 43.1 months). Those experimental subjects included had been treated for ALL at least two months previously. A group of 22 non-neurologically impaired children matched for age and sex served as control subjects. None of the experimental or control subjects had a history of birth trauma, head injury, intellectual impairment, neurological disorder or hearing impairment. Children with genetic diseases were excluded from the study as were experimental subjects with a history of speech and/or language disorders prior to diagnosis of ALL. English was the primary language of all subjects included.

A series of language assessments were used to assess a range of linguistic abilities. The principal language test administered was an age-appropriate measure from the *Test of Language Development* (TOLD) series (Hammill and Newcomer, 1982; Newcomer and Hammill, 1982; Hammill et al., 1987). This series was chosen as all of the tests contain subtests which assess receptive and expressive linguistic abilities in the areas of syntax and semantics. The TOLD-P (primary) was administered to children between the ages of 4;0 and 8;11. The TOLD-I (intermediate) was administered to children between the ages of 9;0 and 11;11. The second edition of the *Test of Adolescent Language* (TOAL-2) was used for subjects between the ages of 12;0 and 18;5. The TOLD-I may be used for children as young as 8;6. However, the TOLD-P was chosen for assessment of Case 7 (aged 8;6) because it offers a variety of both auditory and visual stimulus cues, whereas the TOLD-I is a purely auditory-based test. Similarly, although the TOLD-I may be used for children up to age 12;11, the TOAL-2 was chosen for the assessment of 12-year-olds, because of its greater ability to detect subtle linguistic deficits. The TOAL-2 is composed of subtests assessing grammar and vocabulary skills across reading, writing, listening and speaking modalities. Tables are provided in the TOLD series manuals to convert raw scores for the subtests into standard scores (mean = 10 ± 3). Quotients (mean = 100 ± 15) are composite scores derived from subtest standard scores to specific areas of language impairment, for example, grammar versus vocabulary deficits, or listening versus speaking impairment. All three tests provide an overall language quotient (Spoken Language

Quotient in TOLD-P and TOLD-I; Adolescent Language Quotient in TOAL-2), as well as quotients for listening and speaking. In addition to these quotients, both the TOLD-P and TOLD-I have semantic and syntactic quotients, whilst the TOAL-2 has reading, writing, vocabulary and grammar quotients.

In conjunction with one of the TOLD series tests, the children were all assessed with three other tests. The *Token Test* (DeRenzi and Faglioni, 1978) was administered to children aged 12 years and older, whereas children younger than 12 years of age were assessed with The *Token Test for Children* (DiSimoni, 1978). These tests were selected to detect high-level comprehension deficits. The *Boston Naming Test* (BNT) (Kaplan et al., 1983), and the timed subtests (i.e. Subtest 7: Word Series, Subtest 8: Confrontation Naming, and Subtest 9: Word Association) of the *Clinical Evaluation of Language Function* (CELF) (Semel and Wiig, 1982) were also administered. These assessments of semantic ability were included because semantic skills, particularly word retrieval abilities, have been known to be affected by diffuse brain lesions in groups such as children with closed head injury (Jordan et al., 1988) and children after irradiation (Hudson et al., 1989).

With regard to the CELF subtests, there were varying numbers of children used in the comparison groups for each parameter. The Confrontation Naming Subtest yields two scores: the number of items correct, and the minus time (the time taken to complete the task, subtracted from 120 seconds). However, only children in Grade 3 and above are expected to obtain a minus time score. Therefore, mean minus time scores for the Confrontation Naming Subtest of the CELF are calculated for 18 subjects and their controls, Cases 1–4 inclusive having been omitted. Mean number correct scores were obtainable for 21 subjects, since Case 1 did not have adequate colour knowledge to complete the task.

The findings of the study carried out by Buttsworth et al. (1993) based on performance on the TOLD series of language tests confirmed the preliminary results reported by Jackel et al. (1990) that children treated for leukaemia have impaired language abilities compared to control subjects. In the group of nine children whose ages were greater than 12 years (assessed with the TOAL-2), Buttsworth et al. (1993) observed particularly large discrepancies between the means recorded for the leukaemic and control group for Expressive Language, Grammar and Writing Quotients, the children treated for leukaemia scoring significantly lower quotients than the control subjects. These authors also observed moderate differences between the mean scores achieved by all 22 leukaemic subjects compared to controls for the Overall Language Quotient and Speaking Quotient, and all other measures on the TOAL-2. Although the differences between the mean scores on the remaining subtests of the TOLD-P and TOLD-I were not as large, Buttsworth et al.

(1993) reported that the scores obtained by the leukaemic children on all subtests of all TOLD series assessments were significantly lower than those obtained by their control subjects.

Buttsworth et al. (1993) reported that the ability of the older children treated for leukaemia included in their study to follow spoken commands (as measured by the *Token Test*) was also significantly lower than their controls, a result which concurs with the findings of Taylor et al. (1987). A similar result, however, was not found for the younger children treated for ALL who were assessed on the *Token Test for Children*.

Naming ability was assessed by Buttsworth et al. (1993) using the BNT. They found that the ALL group had a significantly lower mean BNT score than their control subjects. Taylor et al. (1987) who used the Expressive One Word Picture Vocabulary Test (like the BNT a picture naming test), however, failed to find a significant difference in the ability to name between ALL subjects and their healthy siblings. Unlike Jackel et al. (1990) and Taylor et al. (1987) no problem was observed by Buttsworth et al. (1993) to be present in their leukaemic group with regard to confrontation naming and word fluency as measured by the timed subtests of the CELF. The disparity between the findings of Buttsworth et al. (1993) and the results of Taylor et al. (1987) may lie in the different assessment tools. Taylor et al. (1987) used the Stroop Colour Test and the Word Fluency Test from the *Spreen–Benton Aphasia Test* (Gaddes and Crockett, 1975) to assess confrontation naming and word fluency, respectively. Alternatively, the use of different control groups (age- and sex-matched by Buttsworth et al. (1993); sibling control subjects in the study by Taylor et al. (1987) may be reflected in the difference in naming skills.

The disparity between the results obtained by Buttsworth et al. (1993) for the BNT compared with the subtests of the CELF could be due to the nature of the naming tasks involved. The BNT is a confrontation naming task that draws on the subject's existing vocabulary, and on their ability to search for, find and generate the target word if it is present in their vocabulary. The Confrontation Naming Subtest of the CELF, although it is also a convergent task, does not explore vocabulary since there are only seven target words (red, blue, black, yellow, circle, square, triangle), but requires rapid recognition of the stimulus, selection of, and production of the appropriate label for the stimulus item. The Word Association Subtest of the CELF, unlike the previous two naming tasks is a divergent task and needs different semantic–lexical abilities for its successful completion (e.g. generation of many items within a semantic category, determining the category boundaries, rejecting items outside the category).

Expression and Reading Comprehension was found by Taylor et al. (1987) to be deficient in ALL subjects compared with their siblings;

similarly, Waber et al. (1990) found Reading and Spelling (assessed by the Wide Range Achievement Test) in both male and female ALL subjects to be lower than normative test data expectations. This agrees with the low scores on Reading, Writing and Written Language Quotients reported by Buttsworth et al. (1993).

Although the findings of the study carried out by Buttsworth et al. (1993) are suggestive of a link between the treatment process and the occurrence of language disorders in children treated for ALL, it is not possible to attribute the language impairment to a single cause such as the radiotherapy and/or the chemotherapy used in the treatment of this condition. As pointed out in Chapter 3, radiotherapy has been identified as a possible cause of linguistic deficits in children treated for brain tumours (Hudson et al., 1989). Radiation dosage following surgery for brain tumours, however, is much greater (5000–6000 rads) (Marks et al., 1981; Curnes et al., 1986) than the doses used for childhood ALL (1800 or 2400 rads). The findings of Buttsworth et al. (1993) do, however, suggest that even low levels of radiation may contribute to language deficits in some children.

Other than CNS prophylaxis involving cranial irradiation, with or without IT therapy, the other risk factor most often implicated in neuropsychological problems in children treated for ALL is the patient's age at the time of CNS prophylaxis (Ochs and Mulhern, 1988). Buttsworth et al. (1993), however, were unable to demonstrate a correlation between age at diagnosis or radiation dosage and language quotients achieved on the TOLD series by their cohort of children treated for ALL. They cautioned, however, that their sample size was small and that the treatment protocols used on their 22 leukaemic subjects were heterogeneous. The children assessed in their study ranged from patients treated in the 1970s to those whose treatment finished in the early 1990s, leading to differences in the treatment protocols used. In addition, as pointed out by Bleyer (1990), by the early 1990s advances in the diagnosis and treatment of ALL had made it possible to tailor therapy to the individual needs of subgroups of patients, rather than using the same treatment on every patient with ALL. A number of other researchers have considered the effect of age at diagnosis and dosage of cranial irradiation on neuropsychological abilities. Several investigators have reported that younger children (below five years of age) treated for ALL have more severe neuropsychological after-effects than older children (Jannoun, 1983; Moore et al., 1986; Said et al. 1987). Moore et al. (1986) attributed this to enhanced vulnerability of the brain to biological insults during the period of rapid development (Dobbing, 1968). Others, however, did not find this effect (Whitt et al., 1984; Jackel et al., 1990). Tamaroff et al. (1982) found no difference in the cognitive effects of cranial irradiation with doses of 2400 and 1800 rads. According to Said et al. (1987), neuropsychological outcome is better following the reduced dose of 1800 rads of cranial irradiation, if distinct treatment protocols are compared and large numbers of cases are considered. The effects of age at treatment, sex of the subject and dosage of cranial irradiation on language outcome in leukaemic children, as well as the relationship between their cognitive and language abilities, requires ongoing investigation utilizing a large pool of subjects treated with similar protocols.

In addition to language difficulties, some of the children treated for ALL examined by Buttsworth et al. (1993) also had academic difficulties. Of the 12 younger children in their group who were attending primary school, two were experiencing difficulty and had repeated grades. Five of the nine older children had academic problems, especially in Mathematics and English. Difficulties reportedly became more noticeable in secondary school. Academic performance has received consideration in the ALL literature. The *Wide Range Achievement Test* (WRAT) (Jastak and Jastak, 1978), which considers reading, spelling and arithmetic, has been frequently used to measure academic performance of ALL subjects and controls. Significantly poorer WRAT outcomes have been reported for leukaemic patients than their siblings (Taylor et al., 1987) and solid tumour control subjects (Copeland et al., 1985; Moore et al., 1986; Waber et al., 1990). Studies that have compared the WRAT results of leukaemic subjects who had received cranial irradiation with those of subjects who had received prophylaxis consisting of drug therapy only, have not identified significant differences between these two treatment groups (Whitt et al., 1984; Copeland et al., 1985; Ochs et al., 1986).

In summary, the findings of group studies reported to date indicate that language deficits may occur in children subsequent to treatment for ALL. Clinicians need to be aware of the possibility of language impairment as part of the late effects of treatment, so that such children can receive early remediation in areas of deficit, and thus maintain the highest quality of life possible. Routine language assessment of each individual may not be possible (or even necessary) in a busy clinic, but early detection and intervention should be a realistic goal.

Language impairments following treatment for leukaemia: evidence from case studies

Although the findings of Buttsworth et al. (1993) indicated that, as a group, children treated for leukaemia have significant language deficits compared to control subjects, when examined individually it is apparent that the language abilities of the children treated for ALL included in their study varied considerably from individual to individual. Some of the leukaemic subjects demonstrated normal (or in one case above average) language abilities while others had significant language problems. In addition, the performance of the leukaemic subjects on specific language tasks varied widely. Although some of the children treated for ALL demonstrated one or two particularly weak (or strong) areas of language ability that functioned to depress (or elevate) their overall language score, other subjects showed a relatively consistent performance across all language areas. Consequently, it was felt by Buttsworth et al. (1993) that by presenting their data on a group basis only, that important information concerning the variety of language outcome following treatment for ALL may have been lost. As a follow-up to their earlier study, therefore, Murdoch et al. (1994) examined the language abilities of the same children treated for ALL (with the addition of one further child) on an individual basis to enable any observed language problem to be described and discussed with reference to individual variables relating to personal details, medical history, treatment factors etc. Case reports relating to the 23 subjects examined by Murdoch et al. (1994) appear below. For each case, the language tests administered were the same as those outlined above for Buttsworth et al. (1993).

Case reports

Case 1 (Joanne)

Joanne was diagnosed with acute lymphoblastic leukaemia at the age of 2;4. IT MTX (together with other, non-intrathecal drugs) was administered as induction therapy. CNS prophylaxis consisted of IT MTX, vincristine and 6-mercaptopurine. No radiotherapy was administered. MTX was administered both intrathecally and systemically (together with other cytotoxic drugs) for maintenance therapy. Treatment ceased after 26 months, when the subject was aged 4;6. At the time of language assessment, 6 months after completion of treatment, Joanne presented as a lively, outgoing 5-year-old girl who was attending and enjoying pre-school.

Joanne achieved below average scores on the TOLD-P in the subtests of receptive semantics (Picture Vocabulary) and syntactic comprehension (Grammatic Understanding). Scores for the other subtests of the TOLD-P were within the average expected for her age, although the scores for expressive syntax (Sentence Imitation) and auditory discrimination (Word Discrimination) were at the lower end of the normal range. Joanne obtained a below average Overall Language Quotient, and below average quotients for Listening and Semantics. The other language quotients were in the average range. Her Overall Score of 489 on the *Token Test for Children* was more then 2 SD below the age mean of 500 and reinforced the indication of poor syntactic comprehension. The fact that Joanne had difficulty distinguishing between the labels 'yellow' and 'green', however, no doubt contributed to the low score.

The errors she made, though, were not solely a result of this lack of colour knowledge, as they also included shape errors (i.e. circle versus square) and prepositions as well.

Of the three CELF subtests selected it was not possible to administer Confrontation Naming, since this subtest requires the child to be capable of generating the colour and shape of 36 items, and Joanne could not consistently name colours. She knew five of the days of the week required in the Producing Word Series, and thus performed above criterion in comparison to normative data provided in the test manual. The score achieved in Producing Word Associations was also above criterion.

Joanne performed poorly on the BNT correctly naming only 15 out of the 60 items. This score was considerably lower than the mean of 29.6 achieved by the group of five-year-old children tested by Kaplan et al. (1983). Overall, the language tests indicated that Joanne had a mild language impairment, with particular difficulties being experienced in the areas of expressive and receptive semantics and syntactic comprehension. As Joanne had only recently commenced pre-school, there was an insufficient history on which to judge the presence of any academic difficulties. Consequently, it is difficult to gauge whether the depressed language scores represent a language delay that may eventually 'catch up' to normal development, or an impairment that will remain as Joanne matures. As the treatment for ALL began at an age when Joanne would be expected to be acquiring language, it may be that the intensive chemotherapy has slightly delayed the acquisition of normal language skills, rather than actively impairing her existent language abilities.

Case 2 (Greta)

Greta was a girl aged 5;11. Diagnosis of ALL was made at the age of 1;9 and treatment commenced immediately. IT MTX was administered as part of the induction of remission. CNS prophylaxis consisted of a total dose of 1800 rads of radiation, as well as IT MTX, vincristine, cyclophosphamide and ara-C. Maintenance treatment ran for 20 months, and included systematic (but also IT) administration of MTX. Greta was aged 3;8 when maintenance therapy ceased. At the time of language assessment 27 months later, Greta presented as a co-operative, though timid girl, who was enjoying Grade 1 at school.

All subtests and quotients of the TOLD-P were within the normal range. Greta's Overall Score on the *Token Test for Children* was normal for her age with all subtests, except one, being within 1 SD of the mean. The exception was Part 4, where Greta seemed to experience a lapse of concentration, which she regained for the fifth subtest after encouragement from the examiner.

The Producing Word Series and Confrontation Naming Subtests of the CELF were above criterion. The Producing Word Associations Subtest fell below criterion. As all the items generated were good examples of the given category, the limited number of category members generated could have been the result of shyness, rather than word retrieval problems or vocabulary restrictions.

Greta scored 23 (out of a possible 60) on the BNT. According to the 'norms' provided in the test manual, the age-expected score is 29.6. Twenty-nine of the 60 items were simply unknown to Greta, which is not unexpected in a five-year-old child. Of the items that Greta attempted to name, the errors were mainly semantic (e.g. *boat, sailboat* for 'canoe') or perceptual (e.g. *pencil* for 'dart'). Naturally, in a five-year-old, these errors are more indicative of intelligent guessing than of a word-finding problem, as they would be in an adult.

At a time more than two years after cessation of treatment for ALL, Greta's language was found to be developing normally. Academic performance was difficult to gauge, as she had only been attending her first year of school for three months.

Greta was less than two years old at the time of diagnosis (and therefore CNS prophylaxis). Children under five years of age are thought to be most vulnerable to the effects of CNS prophylaxis (Eiser and Lansdown, 1977). As cognitive deficits associated with prophylactic CNS chemotherapy may not manifest until several years after diagnosis (e.g. Pfefferbaum-Levine et al., 1984: Rubenstein et al, 1990; Brown et al., 1992), it would be necessary to monitor Greta on a long-term basis in order to be satisfied that CNS prophylaxis has left no legacy of language impairment.

Case 3 (Nicola)

Nicola was diagnosed with ALL at the age of 2;11. Following induction, she received a radiation dosage of 1800 rads (given in 12 fractions) and IT MTX as part of CNS prophylaxis. There was a slight problem establishing an appropriate dosage in the maintenance stage of treatment owing to drug toxicity. Nicola received approximately 75% of the recommended dosage. Treatment was completed at the age of 4;8, 21 months after ALL was diagnosed. Nicola's language was assessed when she was aged 6;4, 20 months after completion of treatment. She presented as an outgoing child with a cheerful interest in the world, who was enjoying Grade 1 at school.

Nicola obtained scores within the normal range on all subtests and quotients of the TOLD-P. Both the Overall and the individual subtest scores of the *Token Test for Children* were at or above the age-expected mean; indeed, Nicola obtained a score of 507 for Part 4, which was greater than 1 SD above the mean for normal subjects. The three CELF subtests were above criterion. The score of 30 achieved on the BNT was in accord with the published mean of 29 expected for her age. In addition, it compared favourably with the score of 31 achieved by an age- and sex-matched control. In summary, Nicola's language ability was found to be competent and well within the normal limits for her age.

Case 4 (Mark)

Mark was admitted to hospital with a diagnosis of ALL at the age of 3;8. CNS prophylaxis included a radiation dose of 1800 rads. Treatment was completed 24 months later when he was aged 5;8. At the time of language assessment, Mark was aged 7;1, and had been in complete continuous remission for 17 months. He was in Grade 2 at the local primary school, and appeared to be coping satisfactorily. His mother was of the opinion that he was lacking in concentration; this problem had not been reported by his teacher. In addition, his mother felt that Mark was 'not as bright' as he had been prior to the treatment for ALL. Mark presented as a friendly boy who co-operated cheerfully for all tasks.

Mark obtained below average scores on the TOLD-P in the subtests of receptive semantics (Picture Vocabulary) and phonology (Word Articulation). Receptive syntax (Grammatic Understanding) was at the lower end of the average range, whilst the other subtests were in the average range, some at the higher end of the average range, which resulted in a wide variety of quotients. Mark obtained average Overall, Speaking, Semantic and Syntax Quotients and a below average Listening Quotient.

Despite the below average listening skills demonstrated in the TOLD-P, Mark's scores on the *Token Test for Children* were all within the normal range for both age and grade. All three subtests of the CELF were above criterion. Mark achieved a score of 36 on the BNT, which was close to the published 'mean' of 37 expected for children in Grade 2.

With one exception, Mark's language skills were average for his age. The exception was the below average Listening Quotient he obtained on the TOLD-P. This quotient was arrived at by combining the results of the receptive semantics and receptive syntax subtests, both of which were low. Since his ability to follow multi-step spoken instructions was average, an explanation was sought to reconcile the apparent disparity between different listening tasks and scores. Both of the TOLD-P tasks were picture pointing tasks, where the examiner names a stimulus word (for semantics) or sentence (for syntax), and the subject selects one out of a choice of four (or for syntax, three) pictures. Thus, the child must process the visual information (from the pictures) in order to correctly select the match for the auditory information supplied by the examiner. It may be that Mark was too anxious to point to a picture, and was not allowing sufficient time to process both the visual and auditory information in order to make the correct response for these tasks.

Case 5 (Luke)

Luke was diagnosed with ALL at the age of 4;7. The CNS prophylactic stage of therapy included a radiation dosage of 1800 rads. Maintenance therapy was completed 24 months after ALL was diagnosed, when Luke was aged 6;7.

The language test battery was administered when Luke was aged 7;8, 13 months after treatment for ALL had been discontinued. He was in complete continuous remission, and was attending a local church school where he was repeating Grade 1. He was on a waiting list to be seen by a speech/language pathologist, and his mother was anxious for him to receive some form of specialist assistance. Luke presented as a quiet child, who co-operated for all tasks. His ability to concentrate on the tasks seemed limited, but could be regained by an encouragement to keep attending.

Luke achieved below average scores on the TOLD-P in the subtests of expressive syntax (Sentence Imitation and Grammatic Completion), auditory discrimination (Word Discrimination) and phonology (Word Articulation). The other three subtests were within the normal range, although receptive syntax (Grammatic Understanding) was at the lower end of the normal range. Consequently, Luke obtained a below average Overall Language Quotient and below average quotients for Speaking and Syntax. Other language quotients were within normal limits.

Luke performed poorly on the *Token Test for Children*, with only one subtest (Part 1) falling within the normal range expected for his age. The other four subtests and the Overall Score were 2 or more SDs below the age-expected mean. Parts 3 and 5 were 2 SDs below the mean, Part 4 was 3 SDs below the mean, the Overall Score was 4 SDs below the mean, and Part 2 was greater than 4 SDs below the mean. These low scores would appear to reflect the findings of poor auditory memory reported in the neuropsychological tests. It was interesting to note that Luke did not utilize any strategies, such as verbal repetition of the examiner's instruction, to assist him in carrying out the instruction.

Luke achieved a score of 36 on the BNT, which was comparable with the published age-expected mean of 27. The BNT score, taken in conjunction with the two vocabulary subtests of the TOLD-P (where Luke's scores were average) would suggest that his vocabulary and naming ability are normal for his age. However, the Confrontation Naming Subtest of the CELF was below criterion indicating that speed of naming may be slower than average. The other two subtests of the CELF were above criterion.

Luke's language skills were below the normal expectation for his age, with the exception of semantic ability, which was average. The disparity between his average Listening Quotient on the TOLD-P (made up of the Picture Vocabulary and Grammatic Understanding Subtests) and his low scores on the *Token Test for Children* may lie in the differences in the tasks involved. The two TOLD-P subtests involve picture-pointing, with a one in three or one in four chance of the correct answer, whereas the *Token Test for Children* requires a correct action to be made in response to instructions of increasing length and complexity.

Luke's pattern of language deficits seems to be similar to the pattern of language deficits reported by Taylor et al. (1987), who compared leukaemic subjects with their healthy siblings, and found that the leukaemic subjects performed less well than their siblings on tasks requiring speed and accuracy (such as word fluency and contingency naming) and on tasks requiring the ability to follow multiple element directions (*Token Test*). Although Luke's word fluency (Producing Word Associations Subtest of the CELF) was above criterion, the other findings agree with his language deficits.

Case 6 (Thomas)

Thomas was diagnosed with average risk ALL at the age of 2;3. Induction therapy included IT MTX, and CNS prophylaxis included a radiation dosage of 1800 rads and IT MTX. Thomas' treatment was completed 24 months after diagnosis, when he was aged 4;3. Language was assessed at the age of 7;11. He presented as a friendly, outgoing child who was happy to co-operate with all tasks.

All subtests and quotients of the TOLD-P were within the normal range. Similarly, all parts and the Overall Score for the *Token Test for Children* were within 1 SD of the age-expected mean. Thomas achieved a score of 35 on the BNT, which was within 1 SD of the age-expected mean of 37, though considerably lower than the score of 47 achieved by the age- and sex-matched control subject, whose naming ability was above average. The three subtests administered from the CELF were all above criterion. In summary, the results of Thomas' language assessment were consistent with normal language development.

Case 7 (Anita)

Anita was diagnosed with ALL at the age of 5;10. She received 1800 rads of radiotherapy as part of her CNS prophylaxis. Treatment was completed 26 months later, when Anita was aged 8;0. At the time of language assessment, Anita was aged 8;5, and had been in complete continuous remission for 18 months. She presented as a vivacious, co-operative child, who was enjoying Grade 3 at school.

Anita obtained average or above average scores on all subtests and quotients of the TOLD-P. Although most of the subtest scores were in the upper end of the average range, the scores for receptive and expressive syntax (Grammatic Understanding and Sentence Imitation) were greater than 1 SD above the mean, and so were in the above average range.

Scores obtained on the *Token Test for Children* were within or greater than 1 SD of the mean expected for her age. All three subtests of the CELF were above criterion. Anita obtained a score of 41 on the BNT which was within 1 SD above the mean of 38.4 expected for her age. Overall, Anita's language abilities were normal or above average for her age.

Case 8 (Julia)

Julia was aged 3;11 when a diagnosis of ALL was made. She fell into the low risk ALL prognostic group, a 'group of patients [who] do not appear to require cranial radiotherapy nor an intensive consolidation and reinduction phase of treatment'. Consequently, IT MTX was administered as part of Julia's induction, and CNS prophylaxis consisted of IT MTX alone. Treatment was completed when Julia was aged 5;11. Julia's language was assessed when she was aged 8;6 and had been in complete continuous remission for 31 months. She presented as a rather quiet child, who appeared to concentrate well during the lengthy 90-minute session. She was in Grade 3 at school.

Julia's Overall, Speaking, Semantics and Syntax Quotients obtained on the TOLD-P were average, though low average. The Listening Quotient of 70 was below average, as a result of an extremely low receptive semantics score. The scores Julia achieved on the subtests of the TOLD-P varied considerably. The score for receptive semantics (Picture Vocabulary) was greater than 1 SD below the mean. The other subtests were within the average range, though receptive and expressive syntax (Grammatic Understanding and Grammatic Completion) were at the lower end of the average range, whereas expressive semantics was at the upper end of the average range.

All scores of the *Token Test for Children* were within 1 SD of the mean. Julia performed above criterion on all three CELF subtests. Her BNT score of 22 was low in comparison to her expected age norm of 38.

With one exception, Julia's language abilities were normal for age. In light of her poor performance on both the picture vocabulary task of the TOLD-P and a picture naming task (BNT), it would seem that her limited vocabulary, rather than her ability to access names or her listening skills is the chief cause of the low scores. The picture vocabulary task only required the ability to retain one spoken word, and as Julia's scores on the *Token Test for Children* were consistent with good ability to listen and follow multi-element directions, it is unlikely that an impairment in auditory retention ability could have contributed to the low scores achieved on the BNT and the Picture Vocabulary Subtest.

Case 9 (Henry)

Henry was diagnosed with ALL at the age of 3;6. The CNS prophylactic phase of his treatment included 1800 rads of radiotherapy. Maintenance therapy was completed approximately 24 months later when Henry was aged 5;6. At the time of language assessment, 3 years seven months after cessation of treatment, Henry was aged 9;1 and was in Grade 2 at a local primary school, where he had repeated Grade 1. His mother stated that he was very self-conscious of having repeated a grade. Henry was being assessed at a Child Guidance Clinic as a result of learning problems and features of Attention Deficit Disorder (ADD), for which he was taking 20 mg of ritalin daily. In addition to attending the regular classroom Henry was also receiving remedial reading assistance at school, and was on a speech therapy waiting list. Overall Henry presented as a talkative boy, who appeared anxious to perform well. He was slightly built and small for his age. He co-operated willingly, though at times he interrupted inappropriately.

Henry achieved a below average score on the TOLD-I subtest of expressive syntax (Word Ordering). Scores on the other subtests were average. He obtained a below average Syntax Quotient. The other quotients and the Overall Language Quotient were within normal limits.

Henry achieved average scores for Parts 1 and 2 of the *Token Test for Children*. The other three subtests (of increasing length and complexity) and the Overall Score were all greater than 1 SD below the mean expected for his age. Of the three CELF subtests administered, Confrontation Naming was performed above the published criterion. Henry could not name and correctly order the days of the week or the months of the year to complete the Producing Word Series task, and could not generate a sufficient number of foods and animals in the Producing Word Associations task. Henry obtained a score of 29 on the BNT, which was below the test norm for his age.

Overall, the language tests indicated that Henry had a mild language impairment, with particular difficulties being experienced in the areas of expressive and receptive syntax and in high-level language skills.

With regard to the poor score achieved on the Word Ordering Subtest of the TOLD-I, it may be that as the TOLD-I is purely auditorily based, Henry's apparent difficulty in retaining auditory information may have contributed to his poor performance. However, examination of the items on the other syntax subtests would suggest that Henry's syntactic ability is also limited, independent of auditory retention problems. In an appraisal of research findings into the effects of CNS prophylaxis in children with ALL, Chessells (1985) found both auditory learning and memory and attention problems to be two of the cognitive deficits in these children. The question also arises as to the relationship between the ALL treatment and the ADD that was suspected in Henry. There is insufficient information to determine whether the ADD was present before the diagnosis of ALL was made when Henry was three years old, whether the ADD was a result of the CNS prophylaxis, or whether the ADD had developed independent of any prophylactic or chemotherapeutic treatment. The matter is further complicated by the fact that, according to Cousens et al. (1990) the deficits of speed of processing, short-term memory and visual processing evident in ALL survivors and ADD children are similar.

Case 10 (Jenny)

Jenny suffered from seizures at the age of 5 weeks. She was treated with phenobarbitone for 12 months. There was no recurrence of seizures and she developed completely normally. At the age of 3;4 Jenny was admitted to hospital with a diagnosis of ALL. CNS prophylaxis included both 1800 rads of radiotherapy and IT MTX. IT MTX was also administered in a reinduction–reconsolidation phase that occurred after CNS prophylaxis. Treatment was completed 24 months after diagnosis, when Jenny was aged 5;4. At the time of her assessment, Jenny was aged 9;2 and had been in complete continuous remission for 3 years 10 months. She was in Grade 4 at school, and although 2 years previously she had experienced difficulty with peer relationships at school (according to medical file notes), she now stated that she was enjoying school. She presented as a well-mannered child who co-operated cheerfully in all tasks.

All subtests and quotients of the TOLD-I were within the normal range. All subtests and the Overall Score of the *Token Test for Children* were within 1 SD of the range expected for her age. Jenny's scores on the three CELF subtests were above criterion. She achieved a score on the BNT of 34, which was lower than the published mean expected for her age of 41.6. Since most of the errors on the BNT were 'don't know' responses (as opposed to repeated attempts to name the item), the low score obtained by Jenny may reflect vocabulary limitations rather than naming problems and word-finding difficulty. Overall, Jenny's language abilities were within the normal range expected for her age.

Case 11 (Louise)

Louise was admitted to hospital at the age of 4;3 with a diagnosis of ALL. Induction therapy included IT MTX. CNS prophylaxis consisted of IT MTX only, with no radiotherapy administered as Louise was in a favourable prognostic group. Maintenance therapy also included five doses of IT MTX. Treatment was completed 25 months after diagnosis, when Louise was aged 6;4. At the time of language assessment, Louise was aged 9;6 and had been in complete continuous remission for 3 years 3 months. She presented as a friendly, co-operative child who was enjoying Grade 4 at school.

All subtests and quotients of the TOLD-I were within the average range. All subtests and the Overall Score achieved on the *Token Test for Children* were within the normal range expected for her age. The three

CELF subtests were above the normative criteria. Louise obtained a score of 28 on the BNT, which was considerably lower than the published mean score for her age group of 41.6. As Louise achieved above criterion scores and demonstrated no word-finding difficulty on the other naming tasks requiring speed and accuracy (i.e. CELF Subtests 8 and 9), it may be assumed that the low score on the BNT reflects a limitation in vocabulary rather than in lexical accessing. Overall Louise's performance was consistent with age-appropriate language development.

Case 12 (Bernise)

Bernise was diagnosed with ALL at the age of 3;4. Her treatment included 1800 rads of radiotherapy during CNS prophylaxis. Maintenance therapy was completed 3 years 2 months after diagnosis, when she was aged 6;6. At the time of language assessment Bernise was aged 10;10 and had been in complete remission for 4 years 4 months. She was in Grade 5 at school. Assessment took place at the hospital, where she had come for a routine check-up. She presented as a co-operative, relaxed child, thoroughly at ease in her surroundings.

All subtests and quotients of the TOLD-I were within the average range. Four of the five subtests of the *Token Test for Children* were within the normal range. Part 5 and the Overall Score were both more than 1 SD above the mean. The three subtests of the CELF were above criterion. Bernise achieved a score of 46 on the BNT which was normal for her age (according to the published test mean of 43.2). Overall, Bernise's language abilities were normal for her age.

Case 13 (Malcolm)

Malcolm was diagnosed with ALL at the age of 8;7. The CNS prophylactic stage of treatment included a dosage of 1800 rads of radiotherapy. Treatment was completed 25 months after diagnosis, when Malcolm was aged 10;8. Language assessment took place only 10 weeks later, when Malcolm was aged 10;10. He was in Grade 6 at school. Although his teachers reported that he was not experiencing difficulty, his mother expressed the desire that Malcolm be permitted to repeat Grade 6 the following year, as he was younger than most of the children in his grade, and his mother felt he was not socially ready for Grade 7. Malcolm presented as an alert child who co-operated cheerfully in all tasks.

Malcolm obtained average or above average scores on all five subtests of the TOLD-I. The Semantics Quotient fell in the above average range, and all other quotients were in the average range. All subtests and the Overall Score of the *Token Test for Children* were average for his age. Malcolm performed above the criterion presented in the test manual on all three CELF subtests. He achieved a score of 45 on the BNT which is appropriate for his age (test mean = 43.2). In summary Malcolm's performance on the language tests was consistent with normal language development for his age.

Case 14 (Lucy)

Lucy was diagnosed with poor prognosis ALL at the age of 3;9. CNS prophylaxis consisted of 1800 rads of radiotherapy given in 10 fractions over 2 weeks. Maintenance therapy was interrupted due to neutropoenia, impetigo and secondary lymphadenitis. A second course of maintenance therapy, which commenced a month later proceeded without interruption, and included IT MTX. Lucy had otitis media during treatment, which was treated and subsequently cleared. Treatment for ALL was completed 3 years 4 months after diagnosis, when Lucy was aged 7;2. At the time of language assessment, Lucy was aged 11;5 and had been in complete continuous remission for 4 years 3 months. She was assessed at the hospital, where she had come for a routine check-up, and seemed relaxed and familiar with her surroundings. She presented as a happy, outgoing child, who was currently in Grade 7.

Lucy obtained average or above average scores on all five subtests of the TOLD-I. Her Listening and Semantics Quotients were within normal limits, and her Overall Language, Speaking and Syntax Quotients were above average. All subtests and the Overall Score on the *Token Test for Children* were within normal limits for her age. The three CELF subtests were above criterion. She obtained a score of 50 on the BNT. As the 'norms' published in the BNT test manual did not extend to children beyond the age of 10;6 it was not possible to make any comparison between Lucy's score and the test manual. Overall, Lucy's language was average or above average for her age.

Case 15 (John)

John was admitted to hospital with a diagnosis of average risk ALL at the age of 3;8. CNS prophylaxis included a radiation dosage of 1800 rads. Maintenance therapy included IT MTX every 12 weeks. During maintenance therapy, bilateral grommets were inserted due to concern over recurring ear infections and fears that these infections were becoming chronic. Treatment for ALL was completed 3 years 4 months after diagnosis when John was aged 6;11. At the time of language assessment John was aged 12;3 and had been in complete continuous remission for 5 years 4 months. He was in Grade 7 at school. John co-operated willingly on all tasks.

Most of the quotients of the TOAL-2 fell below the average range, although the quotients for Reading, Written Language and Receptive Language were average. John achieved a score of 32 out of a possible 36 on the *Token Test* which, according to the authors of the test (DeRenzi and Faglioni, 1978), is indicative of 'nil' impairment. All three CELF subtests were above criterion. John correctly named 43 of the 60 items included in the BNT.

John exhibited mildly impaired language ability, with depressed scores being recorded in most areas of language assessed. John took a great length of time to complete all of the subtests of the TOAL-2 that required reading, especially the Reading/Grammar and Writing/ Grammar Subtests. As the TOAL-2 is not a timed test, the average scores achieved by John conceal his slowness in reading. This slowness was not evident in his Reading Quotient of 100, which was his best score on the TOAL-2. Reading aloud was also rather slow and dysfluent.

Case 16 (Vicki)

Vicki was a girl aged 13;3 who had been diagnosed with ALL at age 2;4. The CNS prophylaxis included 2400 rads of cranial radiotherapy and maintenance therapy included IT MTX. During the course of maintenance therapy Vicki developed a large meibomian granulomata in each eye that required surgical attention. At the time of the language assessment, Vicki had been in complete continuous remission for 2 years 4 months. She presented as a quiet, co-operative 13-year-old who was in Grade 8. Vicki reported that she was enjoying English, German and Art. A school report from Grade 2 stated that Vicki was progressing satisfactorily, with no significant difficulties in Mathematics. A school report from Grade 6 depicted her as 'average' to 'attaining a good standard' in most subjects, although, in the area of Mathematics called Application Problems, she showed evidence of difficulty being experienced. Furthermore, the most recent Grade 8 report described her overall achievement in the areas of Mathematics, English, and Social Studies as 'minimal'. The same report described her overall achievement in German, Science and Art as 'adequate'. Comments from teachers included, 'seems to be experiencing difficulty' and 'must ask for help when she needs it'.

Vicki achieved a range of quotients on the TOAL-2. The Listening, Reading, Grammar and Receptive Language Quotients were in the average range. The Speaking, Spoken Language and Written Language Quotients, however, were below average, whereas the Writing, Vocabulary and Expressive Language Quotients were poor. Her Overall Language Quotient was also below average. Of the individual subtests that contributed to these composite quotients, three were poor: Speaking/Vocabulary, Writing/Vocabulary and Writing/Grammar. Vicki achieved a score of 32 on the *Token Test*, which is described as 'nil' impairment. Vicki performed above the criterion for her grade on the Producing Word Series and Confrontation Naming Subtests of the CELF, and below criterion on the Producing Word Association Subtest. She obtained a score of 47 on the BNT. In view of the poor results achieved on the vocabulary subtests of the TOAL-2, the BNT score may reflect vocabulary limitations rather than word-finding difficulty.

In summary, Vicki demonstrated mild–moderate language impair-ments, with the language difficulty being more pronounced in written language. Although reading skills were adequate, writing was poor, as was expressive vocabulary. This difficulty was reflected in school reports, which appear to indicate a downward trend in Vicki's academic ability from an average student to one struggling to cope in certain areas.

Case 17 (Jason)

Jason was a boy aged 13;9. He had been admitted to hospital at the age of 4;8 after a series of blood tests, and was treated for suspected juvenile rheumatoid arthritis. Four days later, a diagnosis of average-risk ALL was made and induction therapy was commenced immediately. CNS prophylaxis included IT MTX and 2400 rads of radiotherapy administered in 13 fractions over two and a half weeks. Maintenance therapy commenced 3 months after diagnosis and continued for almost 3 years, and included IT MTX. During and after treatment for ALL, Jason developed a condition that, 21 months after ALL treatment was completed, was diagnosed as ulcerative colitis. It was considered medically noteworthy that a child cured of ALL developed an auto-immune disease, and it was queried whether there was something fundamentally wrong with Jason's immune system, thus rendering him more susceptible to such conditions, or whether the condition may have arisen in connection with the therapy for ALL. A colectomy was performed when Jason was about 12 years of age, and he was reported to be 'doing well'. Jason also had a history of middle-ear infections as a young child. At the time of language assessment, Jason presented as a well-adjusted, pleasant boy aged 13;9 who had been in complete continuous remission for 6 years. He was assessed at his boarding school, where he was enjoying Grade 8.

Most of the TOAL-2 quotients were within average range, although the Listening, Writing and Grammar Quotients were below average. Similarly, three subtests — Listening/Grammar, Writing/Vocabulary and Writing/Grammar were below average. Jason achieved a score of 36 on the *Token Test*. All three CELF subtests were above criterion. He obtained a score of 47 on the BNT.

Overall, Jason exhibited very mild language deficits in the areas of vocabulary, written grammatical skills and listening skills. In other areas his language appeared to be within normal limits.

Case 18 (Margaret)

Margaret was diagnosed with ALL at the age of 6;7. Her CNS prophylaxis included 1800 rads of cranial radiotherapy (in 15 fractions over 3 weeks), as well as four doses of IT MTX. Maintenance therapy also included IT MTX. A CT scan performed after CNS prophylaxis revealed no shift of midline structures, no evidence of abnormal calcification, and normal ventricles and subarachnoid space. Treatment was completed 3 years 1 month after diagnosis, when Margaret was aged 9;8. Language assessment took place 4 years 2 months later, when Margaret was aged 13;11. She was in complete continuous haematological remission, and was in Grade 8 at school. Margaret presented as a timid, under-confident child with poor eye contact. She co-operated with all tasks, but seemed reluctant to enter into conversation.

With one exception, all quotients on the TOAL-2 were very poor. The Listening Quotient was in the poor range. The poorest three subtests were Reading/Grammar, Writing/Grammar and Writing/Vocabulary. Margaret achieved a score of 32 on the *Token Test*, indicative of nil impairment. Of the three CELF subtests, only Producing Word Series (i.e. days of the week, months of the year) was above criterion. Margaret obtained a score of 34 on the BNT which, according to the test manual, is at an age equivalent of approximately seven years.

Overall, Margaret presented with a severe global language impairment, with particular difficulties being experienced in areas of written language. Her relatively high Listening Quotient of 73 and her performance on the *Token Test* suggest that comprehension of spoken language may be her best area of language ability, although still being below age expectation. She failed to meet criteria in all but the word series subtest of the CELF. Examination of her responses in the Confrontation Naming and Producing Word Associations tasks revealed that all of Margaret's responses were correct, but her speed of responses was too slow to achieve the criterion expected for her age.

Case 19 (Frances)

Frances was aged 15;7. She had been diagnosed with ALL at the age of 7;6. Induction included IT MTX. CNS prophylaxis involved 1800 rads of cranial irradiation in 10 fractions over 2 weeks, and IT MTX. Treatment lasted for 3 years 4 months and ceased when Frances was aged 10;10. At the time of language assessment, Frances had been in complete continuous remission for 4 years 9 months, and was enjoying Grade 10 at school. She expressed a particular interest in Art. Frances presented as a friendly, well adjusted 15-year-old, who co-operated willingly with all tasks.

Most of her TOAL-2 language quotients were below average, with two quotients, the Writing and Grammar Quotients, being poor. For both writing subtests (Writing/Vocabulary and Writing/Grammar), low standard scores of 6 and 5, respectively were obtained. Frances achieved a score of 35 on the *Token Test*, which was within normal limits. Two of the three CELF subtests were above criterion. Producing Word Series was below criterion, as Frances omitted one month of the year. However, this omission could be attributed more to nervousness than ignorance. She obtained a score of 48 on the BNT.

Overall, the language tests indicated that Frances had a mild language impairment, with particular difficulties in written language, and to a lesser extent, syntax.

Case 20 (Ivan)

Ivan was diagnosed with ALL at the age of 8;3. His treatment included 1800 rads of radiotherapy. Treatment lasted 3 years 11 months. Ivan was aged 12;2 when therapy ceased. On assessment, 3 years 10 months after the conclusion of ALL treatment, Ivan presented as a pleasant 16-year-old boy who was in Grade 10 at school. He had not repeated a grade, but was older than his classmates as he had commenced school in a different state of Australia, where the age of school entry was older than in his current residential state. He expressed enjoyment of both school and of his casual job at McDonalds. He enthusiastically discussed his career plans to be an airline pilot when he finished his schooling.

All TOAL-2 quotients were average or above average. Ivan achieved a perfect score of 36 on the *Token Test*. All three CELF subtests were above criterion. He also made no errors on the BNT and obtained a perfect score of 60. Overall, Ivan's language abilities were within the normal range expected for his age.

Case 21 (Sean)

Sean was a 16-year-old male. At the age of 2;8 he was diagnosed with ALL. Treatment included IT MTX and 2400 rads of cranial irradiation. ALL therapy was completed 3 years 3 months after diagnosis when Sean was aged 5;11. A neuropsychological assessment was performed 3 months after the conclusion of treatment, and included the McCarthy Scales of Children's Abilities and the Hull 'B' Test of Word Recognition were administered. Sean was described as a boy of average intelligence who was well adjusted and socially competent for his age. His perceptual-performance skills were better than his skills in the other areas assessed, although all were well within normal limits. At the time of language assessment, Sean had recently turned 16 and had been in remission for 10 years and 1 month. He was in Grade 11 at school and was hoping to become a chef when he left school. A recent school report described his academic achievement as 'high' and 'sound' in all subjects except Maths in Society, which was a 'low achievement'. Sean was a quiet boy who co-operated willingly with all tasks.

Most of the TOAL-2 quotients were more than 1 SD below the mean. Consequently, all TOAL-2 quotients were less than average. The Overall Language Quotient was poor, as were most quotients, although two (Writing and Vocabulary) were below average, and three (Reading, Grammar and Receptive Language) were very poor. Sean obtained a score of 31 on the *Token Test*. Two of the CELF subtests were above criterion, but the Confrontation Naming time was too slow and was, therefore, below criterion. He scored 48 on the BNT.

Assessment of Sean's language abilities 10 years after completion of treatment for ALL revealed moderate impairment, with particular difficulties in the areas of syntax and reading. This contrasts with the neuropsychological assessment immediately following the cessation of

ALL therapy, which found all areas (including word recognition and a verbal scale) to be average. The discrepancy between the two assessment results may suggest, therefore, a deterioration in various neuropsychological functions over the 10-year period, perhaps including language. Long latency before manifestation of neurocognitive problems in children treated for ALL is frequently mentioned in the literature. The late effects of cranial radiation therapy in leukaemia and brain tumour subjects may not emerge as clear neurocognitive deficits until four to five years after treatment commences (e.g. Rubenstein et al., 1990). Many authors warn that there is a need for continued evaluation of cognitive functioning in ALL children who have received either cranial irradiation and IT chemotherapy or CNS prophylactic chemotherapy alone (e.g. Brown et al., 1992) in order to identify and remediate potential detrimental neuropsychological sequelae of treatment.

Case 22 (Mathew)

Mathew was diagnosed with ALL at the age of 6;3. His treatment included 2400 rads of radiotherapy, and was completed 2 years 5 months after diagnosis, when he was aged 8;8. At the time of language assessment, Mathew had been in complete continuous remission for 9 years. He was aged 17;8 and was in his final year of high school. He presented as a confident, outgoing young man who was looking forward to studying music at a tertiary level the following year.

All subtests and quotients of the TOAL-2 were average or above average. Mathew made no errors on the *Token Test* and all CELF subtests were above criterion. He obtained a perfect score of 60 on the BNT. Overall, Mathew's language abilities were within the normal limits for his age.

Case 23 (Walter)

Walter was a male aged 17;9. He had been diagnosed with ALL at the age of 2;7. Induction included IT MTX. Initially, his parents refused to permit radiotherapy, so maintenance therapy was commenced. Ten months later, however, Walter's parents agreed to radiotherapy and he received 2400 rads of irradiation to the cranium and spinal column. Maintenance therapy included IT MTX, cystosine-arabinoside and hydrocortisone. Therapy was completed 4 years 2 months after diagnosis, when Walter was aged 6;10. At the time of language assessment, Walter had been in complete continuous remission for 10 years and 11 months, and was in Grade 12 at school. His parents stated that all of their five children were achieving well academically with the exception of Walter and attributed this difference to the leukaemia treatment. He was assessed over two sessions, and presented as a pleasant 17-year-old who was obtaining 'sound achievements' in all school subjects, although he was struggling with Social Maths. He spoke of plans to work in the area of retail buying when he completed school.

Three of the TOAL-2 quotients (Speaking, Reading and Vocabulary) were average. The Listening Quotient was poor, and the remainder of the quotients, including the Overall Language Quotient, were below average for his age. He achieved a score of 36 on the *Token Test*. Two of the CELF subtests were above criterion; the Confrontation Naming Subtest was below criterion. He obtained a score of 50 on the BNT. In summary, Walter's language evidenced a mild impairment, with particular difficulties being experienced in the areas of listening and writing.

To summarize, 13 of the 23 children treated for ALL described above demonstrated language abilities within normal limits according to the standardized tests administered. Nine of the children exhibited mild or moderate language impairment, and one child demonstrated a severe language impairment. Particularly low test performances were observed in the following areas: expressive semantics; expressive vocabulary; receptive semantics; receptive syntax; expressive syntax; written syntax; listening skills; reading and written language.

Factors influencing language outcome following treatment for leukaemia

As discussed in Chapter 2, several factors have the potential to influence language outcomes, including the type and level of CNS prophylaxis applied, the age at treatment, the time elapsed between treatment for ALL and language assessment and the psychosocial effects (e.g. emotional trauma, behavioural disturbances etc.) of having a life-threatening disease.

It is now a well-recognized fact that the administration of CNS prophylaxis, as well as being responsible for the dramatic increase in the survival rate of children diagnosed with ALL (Boring et al., 1991), also involves the risk of adverse neurological and neuropsychological sequelae. Included in these sequelae is cognitive impairment in long-term survivors (e.g. Eiser, 1978, 1980; Meadows et al., 1981; Moss et al., 1981; Jannoun, 1983; Poplack, 1983; Twaddle et al., 1983; Pfefferbaum-Levine et al., 1984; Whitt et al., 1984; Brouwers et al., 1985; Copeland et al., 1985; Said et al., 1987; Brown et al., 1992). Although most studies have addressed cognitive ability in terms of intellectual function and academic achievement, there is little reason to assume that language function should be spared if intellectual function is not.

Whether CNS prophylaxis can be directly causally linked to impaired neuropsychological abilities is a matter of debate. Cranial irradiation, craniospinal irradiation and IT MTX— alone, and in combination — have been suggested by researchers as the factors causing neuropsychological impairment in children treated for ALL. As Cousens et al. (1988) mention, 'one of the points at issue in the debate over the effect of CNS prophylaxis on cognitive functioning is whether observed (IQ) decrements could be at least partly accounted for by psychosocial effects of cancer' (p. 847). Much research has gone into the psychological effect on a child of various life-threatening diseases. Spinetta and Maloney (1975) indicated that there is a need to evaluate the impact at an emotional level of the long-term stresses experienced both by the child with a potentially fatal disease, and by their family. Although there are undoubtedly stresses suffered, an early held view that certain social experiences of the young child can lead to permanent social or intellectual impairment at a later stage has been questioned (Eiser and Lansdown, 1977).

Developing neurobehavioural systems are vulnerable to insult (Altman, 1975). The age at which treatment commences has been suggested as a factor that may affect neuropsychological test performance because myelin is presumed to be still forming at specific sites in the brains of young children (Yakovlev and Lecours, 1967). According to Brown et al. (1992), the radiotherapy literature (e.g. Stehbens et al., 1984; Moehle and Berg, 1985) and the chemotherapy literature (e.g. Copeland et al., 1988) are discrepant concerning age at diagnosis and its relationship to neurocognitive functioning.

Radiation selectively destroys intermitotic and migrating cells in the CNS, with non-lethal changes involving dendritic structures and biochemical functions also occurring (Hicks and D'Amato, 1978). Waber et al. (1992) reason that it is logical to suspect that, among the effects of CNS treatment which includes radiotherapy, there will occur selective alterations of populations of developing neurones or neuronal processes — such as dendritic or axonal structures — whose vulnerability is maturationally determined. In a meta-analysis of published studies that have used radiotherapy prophylactically for children with ALL, Cousens et al. (1988) found that younger children are more affected than are their older peers.

Of the few existing studies which examine the relationship of age and prophylactic chemotherapy alone on high-level cognitive abilities, three studies (Copeland et al., 1988; Dowell et al., 1989; Brown et al., 1992) found that age at the time of diagnosis is not a predictor of neurocognitive performance for children who receive only chemotherapy as CNS prophylaxis. Contrary to this, however, is the finding of Nitchke et al. (1990) (cited in Brown et al., 1992) who investigated neurocognitive functioning in ALL children who received only chemotherapy. Nitchke et al. (1990) found that 70% of the children under the age of four years exhibited neurocognitive deficits, whereas only 14% of the children aged five years and older exhibited any neurocognitive deficits. Brown et al. (1992) are of the opinion that, at present, the data supporting the theory that younger-onset children sustain greater central-processing deficits than do their older counterparts are equivocal. Certainly, in the study reported by Murdoch et al. (1994) no clear pattern of younger-onset children with worse language ability emerged.

According to Rubenstein et al. (1990), clear neuropsychological deficits following cranial radiotherapy for leukaemia and brain tumours may not emerge until four to five years after the initiation of treatment. Similar findings have been reported in children whose CNS prophylaxis involved only IT and systemic chemotherapy (Brown et al., 1992). These latter researchers found that only those children followed up for several years after treatment showed evidence of specific impairment of higher-order cognitive abilities. Of the children treated for ALL assessed by Murdoch et al. (1994) 13 had completed ALL therapy less than four years previously, and 10 children had completed treatment more than four years prior to language assessment. Whereas only three (33%) of the 10 children whose treatment ceased more than four years previously had no language deficit, 10 (77%) of the 13 subjects treated within the past four years evidenced no language impairment. If then, cognitive deficits associated with CNS prophylaxis do not manifest until several years after prophylaxis, it could be expected that more of the children in the more recently treated group examined by Murdoch et al. (1994) would exhibit language deficits if they were reassessed three or four years later.

The psychosocial outcomes of having a chronic, life-threatening disease is another factor that may influence the language abilities of the children treated for ALL. Research into a range of diseases, however, has suggested that children suffering from chronic illness compare in intellectual ability with normal children. This includes such illnesses as cystic fibrosis, which is a chronic life-threatening illness that requires extensive medical care (e.g. Gayton and Friedman, 1973; Burton, 1974), diabetes mellitus (e.g. Ack et al., 1961), and haemophilia (e.g. Olch, 1971). As Eiser and Lansdown (1977) point out, various forms of deprivation in the young child are not inevitably associated with later impairment, nor is early hospitalization necessarily linked with later behaviour problems (Quinton and Rutter, 1976). The latter authors, however, found that hospitalization is associated with deviant behavioural patterns more often in young children than older ones. Eiser (1980) compared the intellectual abilities of two groups of children with chronic illnesses with those of normal children. The two disordered groups included children treated for ALL and children treated for solid tumours. Thus, a comparison was made between two groups who had both suffered life-threatening disease, received chemotherapy and radiotherapy — the difference being that the ALL group had received radiation to the CNS, whilst the solid tumour group had received radiation to some part of the body other than the CNS. Eiser (1980) reasoned that any differences in psychological outcome between these two groups could be attributed to the use of CNS radiation, and not hospitalization or emotional trauma. Eiser (1980) found that, despite the many factors that could limit the intellectual growth of children treated for a life-threatening cancer, those children with solid tumors demonstrated no intellectual impairment. However, Eiser (1980) found that the leukaemic patients did display learning skills and attainments below those of normal children, and concluded that the combined effect of CNS irradiation and chemotherapy was most likely to be responsible.

Using similar reasoning, Cousens et al. (1990) examined the cognitive abilities of four groups of children: children treated for ALL; their siblings; solid tumour survivors; and a group of children with ADD. Cousens et al. (1990) argued that if the cognitive effect seen in the ALL survivors was partly a psychosocial effect of having cancer, then the solid tumour group should also show a deficit in the relevant areas compared to their own siblings. An absence of deficit was taken to imply that cognitive impairment in ALL was not due to psychosocial effects. Based on the findings of Cousens et al. (1990) and Eiser (1980), it is unlikely, therefore, that the language deficits observed in some of the children treated for ALL by Murdoch et al. (1994) are the products of psychosocial effects of leukaemia.

Meadows et al. (1981) considered emotional problems as a possible aetiology for a decline in IQ in children treated for ALL. They used measures of emotional adjustment (sentence completion, three wishes and animal identification) and found that the ALL children with declines in IQ did not show signs of psychological problems serious enough to produce the dysfunctions measured. Other authors, however, have found it more difficult to dismiss emotional factors as possible contributors to neuropsychological impairment in children with leukaemia (e.g. Twaddle et al., 1983; Whitt et al., 1984). As Twaddle et al. (1983) mention, it is not possible in a retrospective study to identify personality factors and psychosocial factors at home and at school, since all these factors will have been influenced by the effects of being ill and by treatment. Murdoch et al. (1994) acknowledge, that as their study was also retrospective, that like many other ALL researchers, they faced the same dilemma as described by Twaddle et al. (1983), that is, the impossibility of identifying and isolating emotional factors at work on the child with leukaemia during treatment.

Tamaroff et al. (1982) stated that previous research had not properly considered the role of emotional factors, in particular, anxiety, on cognitive functioning in children treated for ALL. Tamaroff et al. (1982) cite a number of authors (Schafer, 1948; Anderson and Anderson, 1951; Glasser and Zimmerman, 1967; Kaufman, 1979) who published clinical investigations focusing on the relationship between emotional factors and the Wechsler Intelligence Tests, and subsequently noted that the subtests that comprise the freedom from distractibility (attention/concentration) and short-term memory factor are also the ones most negatively influenced by anxiety. Thus, according to Tamaroff et al. (1982), the neuropsychological detriments reported by other researchers could be the result, in part, of emotional factors, such as anxiety. In a meta-analysis of 30 published comparisons of ALL survivors with control subjects by a range of investigators carried out by Cousens et al. (1988), the authors concluded that the IQ decrement they observed in children treated for ALL probably had two components: a component thought to be common to all young cancer patients, perhaps emotional, and one attributable to the specific treatment received by ALL subjects. As there were children in the ALL group studied by Murdoch et al. (1994) who were very young at the time of diagnosis (and therefore treatment) of leukaemia, it may be that the observed language impairment in these cases also has two contributing components.

Clinical implications of language disorders in children treated for leukaemia

Based on the findings of group studies and case studies reported in the literature to date, it is apparent that although not mandatory, language disorders may occur in children subsequent to treatment for leukaemia. A large variation in the language abilities of children who have undergone such treatment has been observed, ranging from above normal to severely impaired language function. Although routine assessment of this population by speech and language pathologists does not appear warranted, health professionals, parents, caregivers and teachers of leukaemic children need to be aware of the possibility of children treated for ALL developing language disorders, particularly as part of the long-term effects of treatment. Certainly, there is a need for hospital-based speech-language pathologists to take an educative role with medical and other professionals working in oncology units to alert them to the possible negative linguistic outcomes in children treated for ALL. Further, considering the negative effect of linguistic impairment on later learning and academic achievement, speech and language pathologists working in community and educational settings need to actively educate parents, caregivers and teachers of children treated for leukaemia as to the possible long-term effects of that treatment with a view to encouraging such persons to refer these children for early consultation with relevant professionals.

References

Ack M, Miller I, Weil WB Jr (1961) Intelligence of children with diabetes mellitus. Pediatrics 28: 764–770.

Altman J (1975) Effects of interference with cerebellar maturation of the development of locomotion: an experimental model of neurobehavioural retardation. In

Buchwald NA, Brazier MAB (eds) Brain Mechanisms in Mental Retardation. New York: Academic Press: 41–91.

Anderson HH, Anderson GL (1951) Projective Techniques. Englewood Cliffs, NJ: Prentice-Hall.

Bleyer WW (1990) Acute lymphoblastic leukemia in children: advances and prospectus. Cancer 65: 689–695.

Boring CC, Squires TS, Tong T (1991) Cancer statistics, 1991. CA — A Cancer Journal for Clinicians 41: 19–35.

Brouwers P, Riccardi R, Fedio P, Poplack DG (1985) Long-term neuropsychologic sequelae of childhood leukemia: correlation with CT brain scan abnormalities. Journal of Pediatrics 106: 723–728.

Brown RT, Madan-Swain A, Pais R, Lambert RG, Baldwin K, Casey R, Frank N, Sexson SB, Ragab A, Kamphaus RW (1992) Cognitive status of children treated with central nervous system prophylactic chemotherapy for acute lymphocytic leukemia. Archives of Clinical Neuropsychology 7: 481–497.

Burton L. (ed.) (1974) Care of the Child Facing Death. London: Routledge & Kegan Paul.

Buttsworth DL, Murdoch BE, Ozanne AE (1993) Acute lymphoblastic leukaemia: language deficits in children post-treatment. Disability and Rehabilitation 15: 67–75.

Chessells JM (1985) Cranial irradiation in childhood lymphoblastic leukaemia: time for reappraisal? British Medical Journal 291: 686.

Ch'ien LT, Rhomes JA, Verzosa MS, Coburn TG, Goff JR, Hustu HO, Price RA, Seifert MJ, Simone JV (1981) Progression of methotrexate-induced leukoencephalopathy in children with leukaemia. Medical and Pediatric Oncology 9: 133–141.

Copeland DR, Fletcher JM, Pfefferbaum-Levine B, Jaffe N, Reid H, Maor M (1985) Neuropsychological sequelae of childhood cancer in long-term survivors. Pediatrics 75: 745–753.

Copeland DR, Dowell RE, Fletcher JM, Sullivan MP, Jaffe N, Cangir A, Frankel LS, Judd BW (1988) Neuropsychological test performance of pediatric cancer patients at diagnosis and one year later. Journal of Pediatric Psychology 13: 183–196.

Cousens P, Waters JS, Said J, Stevens M (1988) Cognitive effects of cranial irradiation in leukemia: a survey and meta-analyses. Journal of Child Psychology and Psychiatry 29: 839–852.

Cousens P, Ungerer JA, Crawford JA, Stevens MM (1990) The nature and possible causes of cognitive deficit after childhood leukaemia. Brain Impairment: Advances in Applied Research: Proceedings of the Fifteenth Annual Conference of the Australian Society for the Study of Brain Impairment, 173–181.

Curnes JT, Laster DW, Ball MR, Moody DM, Witcofski RL (1986) MRI of radiation injury to the brain. American Journal of Roentgenology 147: 119–124.

DeRenzi R, Faglioni P (1978) The Token Test. Cortex 14: 41–49.

DiSimoni F (1978) The Token Test for Children. Hingham, MA: Teaching Resources.

Dobbing J (1968) Vulnerable periods in the developing brain. In Davison AN, Dobbing J (eds) Applied Neurochemistry. Oxford: Blackwell.

Dowell RE, Copeland KR, Judd BW (1989) Neuropsychological effects of chemotherapeutic agents. Developmental Neuropsychology 5: 17–24.

Duffner PK, Cohen ME, Thomas PRM (1983) Late effects of treatment on the intelligence of children with posterior fossa tumours. Cancer 51: 233–237.

Duffner PK, Cohen ME, Thomas PRM, Lansky SB (1985) The long-term effects of cranial irradiation on the central nervous system. Cancer 56: 1841–1846.

Eiser C (1978) Intellectual abilities among survivors of childhood leukaemia as function of CNS irradiation. Archives of Disease in Childhood 53: 391–395.

Eiser C (1980) Effects of chronic illness on intellectual development: a comparison of normal children with those treated for childhood leukaemia and solid tumours. Archives of Disease in Childhood 55: 766–770.

Eiser C, Lansdown R (1977) Retrospective study of intellectual development in children treated for acute lymphoblastic leukaemia. Archives of Disease in Childhood 52: 525–529.

Gaddes WH, Crockett DJ (1975) The Spreen–Benton Aphasia tests — normative data as a measure of normal language development. Brain and Language 2: 257–280.

Gayton WF, Friedman SB (1973) Psychological aspects of cystic fibrosis. American Journal of Disease in Childhood 126: 856–859.

Glasser AJ, Zimmerman H (1967) Clinical Interpretation of the WISC. New York: Grune & Stratton.

Hammill DD, Newcomer PL (1982) Test of Language Development — Intermediate. Austin, TX: Pro-Ed.

Hammill DD, Brown VL, Larsen SC, Wiederhold JL (1987) Test of Adolescent Language 2: A Multidimensional Approach to Assessment. Austin, TX: Pro-Ed.

Hicks S, D'Amato CJ (1978) Effects of ionizing radiation on developing brain and behavior. In Gottleib G (ed.) Studies on the Development of Behavior and the Nervous System: Vol. 4. Early Influences. New York: Academic Press: 36–72.

Hudson LJ, Murdoch BE, Ozanne AE (1989) Posterior fossa tumours in childhood: associated speech and language disorders post-surgery. Aphasiology 3: 1–18.

Jackel CA, Murdoch BE, Ozanne AE, Buttsworth DL (1990) Language abilities of children treated for acute lymphoblastic leukaemia: preliminary findings. Aphasiology 4: 45–53.

Jannoun L (1983) Are cognitive and educational development affected by age at which prophylactic therapy is given in acute lymphoblastic leukaemia? Archives of Disease in Childhood 58: 953–958.

Jastak JF, Jastak SR (1978) The Wide Range Achievement Test Manual of Instructions (revised edition). Wilmington: Jastak Associates.

Jordan FM, Ozanne AE, Murdoch BE (1988) Long term speech and language disorders subsequent to closed head injury in children. Brain Injury 2: 179–185.

Kaplan E, Goodglass H, Weintraub S (1983) Boston Naming Test. Philadelphia, PA: Lea & Febiger.

Kaufman AS (1979) Intelligence Testing with the WISC-R, New York: Wiley & Sons.

Marks JE, Baglan RJ, Prassad SC, Blank WF (1981) Cerebral radionecrosis: incidence and risk in relation to dose, time, fractionation and volume. International Journal of Radiation, Oncology, Biology and Physics 7: 243–252.

Meadows AT, Massari DJ, Ferguson J, Gordon J, Littman P, Moss K (1981) Declines in IQ scores and cognitive dysfunctions in children with acute lymphocytic leukaemia treated with cranial irradiation. Lancet ii: 1015–1018.

Meohle KA, Berg RA (1985) Academic achievement and intelligence test performance in children with cancer at diagnosis and one year later. Journal of Developmental and Behavioral Pediatrics 6: 62–64.

Moore IA, Kramer J, Albin A (1986) Late effects of central nervous system prophylactic leukaemia treatment on cognitive functioning. Oncology Nursing Forum 13: 45–51.

Moss HA, Nannis ED, Poplack DG (1981) The effects of prophylactic treatment of the central nervous system on the intellectual functioning of children with acute lymphoblastic leukemia. American Journal of Medicine 71: 47–52.

Murdoch BE, Boon DL, Ozanne AE (1994) Variability of language outcomes in children treated for acute lymphoblastic leukaemia: an examination of 23 cases. Journal of Medical Speech–Language Pathology 2: 113–123.

Newcomer PL, Hammill DD (1982) Test of Language Development — Primary. Austin, TX: Pro-Ed.

Nitchke R, Chaffin M, Bowman M, Wilson D, Sexhauer C (1990) MRI detection of transient leukencephalopathy and neuropsychological findings in children treated for acute lymphocytic leukemia. Paper presented at the Third Annual Meeting of the American Society of Pediatric Hemotology Oncology, Chicago, IL.

Ochs JJ, Mulhern RK (1988) Late effects of antileukemic treatment. Pediatric Clinics of North America 35: 815–833.

Ochs JJ, Berger P, Brecher ML, Sinks LF, Kinkel W, Freeman AI (1980) Computed tomography brain scans in children with acute lymphoblastic leukemia receiving methotrexate alone as central nervous system prophylaxis. Cancer 45: 2274–2278.

Ochs JJ, Parvey LS, Mulhern R (1986) Prospective study of central nervous system changes in children with acute lymphoblastic leukaemia receiving two different methods of central nervous system prophylaxis. Neurotoxicology 7: 217–226.

Olch D (1971) Effects of hemophilia upon intellectual growth and academic achievement. Journal of Genetics and Psychology 119: 668–743.

Peylan-Ramu N, Poplack DG, Pizzo PA, Adornato BT, Dichiro G (1978) Abnormal CT scans of the brain in asymptomatic children with acute lymphocytic leukemia after prophylactic treatment of the central nervous system with radiation and intrathecal chemotherapy. New England Journal of Medicine 298: 815–818.

Pfefferbaum-Levine B, Copeland DR, Fletcher JM, Reid HL, Jaffe N, McKinnon WR (1984) Neuropsychological assessment of long-term survivors of childhood leukemia. American Journal of Pediatric Hematology/Oncology 6: 123–128.

Pizzo PA, Poplack DG, Bleyer WA (1979) Neurotoxicities of current leukaemia therapy. American Journal of Paediatric Haematology and Oncology 1: 127–140.

Poplack DG (1983) Evaluation of adverse sequelae of central nervous system prophylaxis in acute lymphoblastic leukaemia. In Mastrangelo R, Poplack DG, Riccardi R (eds) Central Nervous System Leukemia. Boston, MA: Martinus Nijhoff: 95–103.

Price RA, Birdwell DA (1978) The central nervous system in childhood leukaemia: III. Mineralizing microangropathy and dystrophic calcification. Cancer 42: 717–728.

Quinton D, Rutter M (1976) Early hospital admissions and later disturbances of behaviour: an attempted replication of Douglas' findings. Developmental Medicine and Child Neurology 18: 447–459.

Rubenstein CL, Varni JW, Katz ER (1990) Cognitive functioning in long-term survivors of childhood leukemia: a prospective analysis. Developmental and Behavioural Pediatrics 11: 301–305.

Said JA, Waters BGH, Cousens P, Stevens MM (1987) Neuropsychological after-effects of central nervous system prophylaxis in survivors of childhood acute lymphoblastic leukaemia. In Gates GR (ed.) Proceedings of the Twelfth Annual Brain Impairment Conference. Armidale: Australian Society for the Study of Brain Impairment.

Schafer R (1948) The Clinical Application of Psychological Tests. New York: International University Press.

Semel EM, Wiig EH (1982) Clinical Evaluation of Language Functions. Columbus, OH: Charles E Merrill.

Spinetta JJ, Maloney LJ (1975) Death anxiety in the out-patient leukemic child. Pediatrics 56: 1034–1037

Stehbens JA, Kisker CT, Wilson BK (1984) Achievement and intelligence test–retest performance in pediatric cancer patients at diagnosis and one year later. Journal of Pediatric Psychology 8: 47–56.

Tamaroff M, Miller DR, Murphy ML, Salwen R, Ghavimi R, Nir Y (1982) Immediate and long-term posttherapy neuropsychologic performance in children with acute lymphoblastic leukemia treated without central nervous system radiation. Journal of Pediatrics 101: 524–529.

Taylor HG, Albo VC, Phebus CK, Sachs BR, Bierl PG (1987) Postirradiation treatment outcomes for children with acute lymphocytic leukaemia: clarification of risks. Journal of Pediatric Psychology 12: 395–411.

Tebbi CK (1982) Major Topics in Pediatric and Adolescent Oncology. Boston, MA: GK Hall Medical Publishers.

Twaddle V, Britton PG, Craft AC, Noble TC, Kernahan J (1983) Intellectual function after treatment for leukaemia or solid tumours. Archives of Disease in Childhood 58: 949–952.

Waber DP, Urion DK, Tarbel NJ, Niemyer C, Gelber R, Sallan S (1990) Late effects of central nervous system treatment of acute lymphoblastic leukemia in childhood are sex-dependent. Developmental Medicine and Child Neurology 32: 238–248.

Waber DP, Bernstein JH, Kammerer BL, Tarbell NJ, Sallan SE (1992) Neuropsychological diagnostic profiles of children who received CNS treatment for acute lymphoblastic leukemia: the systemic approach to assessment. Developmental Neuropsychology 8: 1–28.

Whitt JK, Wells RJ, Lauria MM, Wilhelm CL, McMillan CW (1984) Cranial radiation in childhood acute lymphocytic leukemia: neuropsychologic sequelae. American Journal of Disease in Childhood 138: 730–736.

Yakovlev PI, Lecours A (1967) The myelogenetic cycles of regional maturation of the brain. In Minkonski A (ed.) Regional Development of the Brain in Early Life. Oxford: Blackwell: 3–64.

Chapter 7
Discourse abilities of children treated for neoplastic conditions

BRUCE E MURDOCH, DEBORAH L BOON AND
LISA J HUDSON

Introduction

As documented in earlier chapters of this book (see Chapters 3 and 6), language deficits have been identified as one of the adverse sequelae of treatment for various childhood neoplastic conditions including posterior fossa tumours and acute lymphoblastic leukaemia (ALL). The investigations of language disorders described in those chapters relied primarily on standardized language assessments, which focused on the syntactic and semantic aspects of language. More recently, the scope of language assessment has been broadened to encompass not only the structure and meaning of language (i.e. syntax and semantics) but also the use of language in naturalistic contexts (i.e. pragmatics). In particular, in the late 1970s child language research extended its focus from basic rules of sentence formation and simple relational or naming vocabulary to include linguistic units larger than the sentence (Johnston, 1982). These units, referred to as 'discourse units', can be considered as communication acts serving the needs of particular moments and audiences, and involve such situations as conversation, instruction and narrative. Enquiry into language acquisition and use now includes finding out how units of discourse are affected by varying contexts.

With the linguistic focus of child language research extended to include pragmatics, it became evident that children must learn not only how to transform ideas into sentences but also into other aspects of language. Such aspects include: what needs to be said, and in what way, in order to achieve the best communication in a given point of time. Story-telling is a 'natural forum' for such learning (Johnston, 1982). In concurrence with this suggestion, Liles (1987) stated that a speaker's use of narrative is thought to be sensitive to extralinguistic contexts (i.e. the text has a social function) and that it is a challenge to account for the specific contributions of the interacting variables in discourse. One technique that has emerged as a promising method for assessing the multilevel processes used during discourse is analysis of narrative texts (Liles, 1987). According to many authors, (e.g. Rumelhart, 1975; Johnson and Mandler, 1980) discourse units have their own structured rules and guiding principles. These principles (like sentence and word level rules) must be learned and consequently narratives grow more sophisticated with increasing age or developmental level (Umiker-Sebeok, 1979; Klecan-Aker et al., 1987). Johnston (1982) suggested that the learning of discourse rules continues well through the school-age years, and thus, analysis of narrative discourse in older language-disordered children may provide valuable insights into language behaviour. Since children treated for childhood neoplastic conditions have been found to display language deficits in structured language assessments (Buttsworth et al., 1983; Jackel et al., 1990), it may well be that they, like other groups of language-disordered children, may also demonstrate differences in creative narratives when compared to normal children.

There are several procedures available that allow the investigation of various aspects of narrative production. A child's understanding and use of story grammar has been recognized as an important factor in the comprehension and production of narratives (Page and Stewart, 1985; Roth and Spekman, 1986). A story grammar is a set of rules that describes the internal structure of a story. An ideal story is initiated with a setting statement and concludes once a resolution or outcome has been reached.

A narrator's ability to produce a cohesive text that is easily recognized as a meaningful and unified whole can be evaluated using Halliday and Hasan's (1976) description of cohesion in English. Although Halliday and Hasan's (1976) analysis is concerned with the cohesive links or 'ties' between sentences, the means by which the episodes within a story are connected to each other is also an important factor in the production of a well-formed story. Stein and Glenn (1979) specified four possible interepisodic relations: temporal, causal, embedded and simultaneous.

In addition to the evaluation of story grammar knowledge and the use of cohesive devices, researchers have examined narrative samples for syntactic complexity, length, units of content included, and fluency (Hartley, 1986; Ernest-Baron et al., 1987; Roth and Spekman, 1989). Applebee (1978) determined six developmental stages of narrative production. Although it has been claimed that by the age of five to six years, children are able to formulate a true narrative (i.e. the final stage in Applebee's continuum) (Botvin and Sutton-Smith, 1977; Applebee, 1978), there is evidence to suggest that both normally achieving and language-impaired children may not necessarily produce true narratives by six years of age (Olley, 1989).

To date, researchers employing one or more of the above mentioned narrative analyses have differentiated between normally achieving and learning-disabled, language-impaired/delayed and closed head-injured subjects on the basis of qualitative and quantitative measures of narrative performance.

The majority of narrative studies have considered the storytelling abilities of language-impaired or language-delayed children. When compared to age-matched and/or language-matched control groups, many differences in story generation have been determined. Relative to their normally achieving peers, language-impaired/delayed children have been found to: produce significantly shorter stories, generate either primitive narratives or focused chains rather than true narratives, include different story grammar categories in their stories, include more inaccurate, irrelevant and repetitive information, produce a higher proportion of incomplete episodes and demonstrate inappropriate sequencing of events and an inability to tie episodes together using interepisodic relations (Liles, 1985, 1987; Merritt and Liles, 1987; Olley, 1989). Analysis of the cohesive techniques employed by language-impaired children has revealed the use of fewer cohesive devices per utterance, more inappropriate cohesive devices per utterance and a greater proportion of incomplete and erroneous cohesive ties (Liles, 1985, 1987; Olley, 1989).

Although the pragmatic functions of language have been addressed in language-delayed and learning-disabled children (Liles, 1985; Roth and Spekman, 1986; Olley, 1989), a pragmatic orientation to the analysis of language has only been employed by a few researchers in the field of acquired language disorders in children (Dennis, 1980; Jordan et al., 1991; Hudson and Murdoch, 1992; Boon et al., 1994). In particular, only two reported studies have addressed pragmatic abilities in children treated for neoplastic conditions. Hudson and Murdoch (1992) analysed the spontaneously generated narratives of children treated for posterior fossa tumours, whereas Boon et al. (1994) examined the performance of children treated for ALL on creative narrative tasks. The procedures used in these latter two studies, together with their findings, are summarized below.

Procedures for assessing narrative abilities of children treated for neoplastic conditions

In the two reported studies that have investigated the discourse abilities of children treated for neoplastic conditions, the authors determined to elicit typical narratives rather than optimal narratives from their subjects. A typical narrative is one that a child is likely to produce in conversation at home, and in relating to the news of the day etc. In contrast, an optimal narrative is the same child's best narrative. Boon et al. (1994)

and Hudson and Murdoch (1992) believed that typical narratives would give a better representation of the children's day to day production rather than a somewhat artificially advanced optimal narrative. Therefore, original stories were required and a story production task was chosen. In order to maintain some common ground for the purpose of comparison, it was necessary to obtain medium structure narratives, and consequently, Boon et al. (1994) and Hudson and Murdoch (1992) decided to use a figurine with an obvious and definite vocation to elicit the story. Given that violence is a prominent theme in children's narrative (Peterson and McCabe, 1983; Kemper, 1984), the figurine selected was 'GI Joe', a man attired in a military uniform, to provide a topic of violence.

The spontaneously generated narratives were elicited by presenting each of the children treated for posterior fossa tumour with the figurine. The examiner then gave the following instructions: ' I want you to give this man a name and then tell me a story about him — the sort of story you might read or write. It can be a short story or as long as you like'. The narrative produced by each child was audiotaped and later transcribed into standard orthography.

Transcribed narratives were initially segmented by Hudson and Murdoch (1992) into sentences. Halliday and Hasan (1976) defined a sentence as a clause complex: a head clause together with other clauses that modify it. Using this definition as a guideline, more specific rules were devised by Jordan et al. (1991) and used by Boon et al. (1994) and Hudson and Murdoch (1992) to clarify the delineation of sentence boundaries. These rules were employed by Jordan et al. (1991) for the analysis of narratives generated by children with closed head injury. The number of sentences in a narrative served as a measure of story length.

The literature contains reference to a variety of procedures that can be used to analyse narratives. Johnston (1982) outlined four main perspectives on narrative structure: story grammars, scripts, textual cohesive devices and communication acts. Two of these four different views of narratives, story grammars and the textual cohesive devices, were selected by Boon et al. (1994) and Hudson and Murdoch (1992) as analysis procedures for the narratives of children treated for neoplastic conditions. Both procedures have been used in previous research in both normal and impaired populations, and story grammar analysis has been modified specifically by Roth and Spekman (1986) for analysis of narratives of learning-disabled children. Story grammar analysis is also particularly suitable for use with oral spontaneous narratives, such as those elicited by Boon et al. (1994) and Hudson and Murdoch (1992).

A story grammar is a description of the structural regularities in a particular kind of text, best exemplified by folktales and fables from the oral tradition. Story grammars describe the rules governing the structure of a story, and are based on researchers' (e.g. Labov, 1972; Rumelhart,

1975; Mandler and Johnson, 1977) analysis of folktales and children's narratives from many cultures. The procedure for story grammar analysis devised by Stein and Glenn (1979) and subsequently modified by Roth and Spekman (1986) was employed by Boon et al. (1994) and Hudson and Murdoch (1992) to analyse the narratives of their children treated for leukaemia and posterior fossa tumours, respectively. textual cohesive devices are concerned with the linguistic tools used by the speaker to link individual sentences, and thereby create a coherent text. These cohesive devices were detailed by Halliday and Hasan (1976), and have been widely used by researchers. Boon et al. (1994) and Hudson and Murdoch (1992) analysed cohesion using the system developed by Halliday and Hasan (1976) and extended by Liles (1985). In addition to being analysed for story grammar composition and textual cohesion, both studies also assigned each narrative to one of the six developmental stages according to the model devised by Applebee (1978).

Narrative abilities of children treated for posterior fossa tumours

Hudson and Murdoch (1992) elicited and analysed narrative samples from 16 children (11 M; 5 F) treated for posterior fossa tumour using the procedures outlined in the previous section. Their findings demonstrated that the narratives collected from the children treated for posterior fossa tumours did not differ to those collected from a group of age- and sex-matched control subjects on a number of parameters including: story length, number of episodes produced, proportion of complete episodes, structure of episodes, story category usage, number of cohesive ties used per sentence, use of cohesive categories and developmental stage. Overall, the ability of the children treated for posterior fossa tumours to spontaneously generate a novel story did not appear to be greatly affected, an observation that contrasts with reports that children with developmental language deficits perform more poorly than their age- and/or language-matched peers on narrative measures (Liles, 1985, 1987; Merritt and Liles, 1987; Olley, 1989; Swartzlander and Naremore, 1989).

Results for those narrative measures that evaluated the types of interepisodic relation used and cohesive adequacy did, however, show a significant difference between the subjects treated for tumour and their control subjects. Hudson and Murdoch (1992) noted that the two groups differed in their use of the interepisodic relation 'and', in that the children treated for posterior fossa tumours tended to produce episodes that occurred simultaneously (i.e. 'and'). Although the 'and' relation was not used by any member of the control group, it was the second most frequently used interepisodic link employed by the children treated for posterior fossa tumours. This finding differs from the narrative features evidenced in Roth and Spekman's (1986) learning-disabled population who failed to use as many concurrent episodes as the control group. Their learning-disabled subjects also used fewer causal relations than their normally achieving peers. Roth and Spekman (1986) proposed that interepisodic relations involving simultaneous events and direct causality are more complex than the relation that links episodes occurring in a logical temporal order. Closer examination of the narrative samples produced by the children treated for posterior fossa tumours studied by Hudson and Murdoch (1992) revealed that there were, in fact, only six examples of the 'and' relation demonstrated by five of the subjects treated for tumours. Of these examples, four were used when an event or character tangential to the theme or plot was described. One was used incorrectly when a 'then' relation would have been appropriate, and another was used during an incoherent narrative when the character was apparently carrying out activities at the same time. Hence, an 'ideal' example of the 'and' relation was not demonstrated by the subject group and it appears the control group avoided its use altogether. This observation concurs with Roth and Spekman's (1986) claim that linking episodes using 'and' is a complex narrative skill for both normal and impaired children, and limits the value of the significant interepisodic findings obtained by Hudson and Murdoch (1992).

The most significant finding of the study reported by Hudson and Murdoch (1992) related to cohesive adequacy. Their control group evidenced a higher proportion of complete cohesive ties than the group comprising children treated for posterior fossa tumour and, in turn, the latter group used significantly more erroneous ties than their age-matched peers. Both groups were noted to evidence a similar percentage of incomplete ties in their narratives. A reduction in the ability to use complete cohesive ties has frequently been documented in the narratives of learning-disabled and language-impaired children (Liles, 1985; Olley, 1989; Roth and Spekman, 1989). Liles (1985) compared the narratives produced by 20 language-impaired children across two listener conditions. The children related a movie story-line to an adult who had viewed the movie with them (the shared condition), and to an adult who had not seen the movie (the unshared condition). In that Liles' (1985) language-impaired subjects used fewer incomplete ties when telling the story in the unshared listener condition as compared to the shared listener condition, it was proposed that the higher frequency of incomplete and erroneous ties in the narratives of language-impaired children, relative to a group of age-matched control subjects, is due to poor narrative organization, not an inability to recognize a listener's need for information. Liles (1985) also found that both the language-impaired and control groups used a greater percentage of incomplete ties when talking to the informed listener, knowing that the listener was capable of filling in the gaps. The language-impaired children did not, however, alter the percentage of erroneous ties used with the informed and uninformed listeners, suggesting that the presence of erroneous ties is more indicative of cohesive deficiency than incomplete ties. This conclusion is supported by the findings of Hudson and Murdoch (1992) that both the tumour and control children in their study produced the same percentage of incomplete ties but differed in the number of erroneous ties used.

The findings of the study conducted by Hudson and Murdoch (1992) further suggest that cohesive adequacy may be a particularly vulnerable aspect of narrative production. This observation is supported by the robust nature of the other narrative measures investigated. Liles (1985) suggested that the use of erroneous ties may be evidence of reduced verbal ability, and may be brought on by momentary confusion or an increase in contextual complexity. It is also possible that the successful use of cohesive devices is related to syntactic and semantic abilities. Cohesion in a spontaneously generated narrative requires a high level of competence in the use of pronominals, demonstratives, conjunctions and ellipsis, all of which may pose problems for children with syntactic deficits (Bloom and Lahey, 1978; Wiig and Semel, 1984). The use of lexical ties requires a broad semantic knowledge if one is to select vocabulary that will help unify a text. Hence, the reduced syntactic and semantic abilities of children treated for posterior fossa tumours (see Chapter 3), may have affected their ability to use cohesion successfully.

Several factors may have accounted for the limited number of narrative differences between the tumour and control groups observed by Hudson and Murdoch (1992). Firstly, 10 of the subjects underwent tumour excision and central nervous system (CNS) prophylaxis when older than six years of age and hence, had the opportunity to acquire narrative knowledge (and possibly 'true narratives') prior to experiencing cerebral trauma. Narrative skills may have been retained despite the acquisition of semantic and syntactic difficulties as shown by the TOLD series of tests (see Chapter 3). Hudson and Murdoch (1992) found no evidence that age at diagnosis and treatment affected narrative performance, however, they conceded that larger subject numbers would be required to confirm this observation.

Secondly, although as a group the semantic and syntactic abilities of the children treated for posterior fossa tumours were significantly below those of the control group, Hudson and Murdoch (1992) noted that not all of the subjects achieved language scores outside the normal range of performance. Although many achieved low-average language scores, seven of the 16 subjects obtained language scores that were within 1 SD of the Test of Language Development series mean quotient of 100 for normals. Despite claims that narrative analyses are sensitive to aspects of language that standardized tests overlook, these seven subjects may have masked the narrative performance of the nine subjects with poor semantic and/or syntactic skills as determined by traditional language tests.

In summary, the findings of the study conducted by Hudson and Murdoch (1992) indicated that the spontaneously generated narratives of children treated for posterior fossa tumour were similar to those produced by age- and sex-matched control subjects. Cohesive adequacy was the major discourse feature found to be deficient in the narratives of the children treated for posterior fossa tumour. Consequently, the results of the study implied a need to examine the adequacy of cohesive markers utilized by these children. Hudson and Murdoch (1992) indicated the need to investigate the relationship between the types of erroneous cohesive ties produced and the semantic and/or syntactic abilities demonstrated by the children.

Narrative abilities of children treated for acute lymphoblastic leukaemia

Boon et al. (1994) recorded the creative narratives of 23 children (12 M; 11 F) who had undergone CNS prophylaxis for ALL. The procedures used to elicit and analyse the narratives were the same as those used by Hudson and Murdoch (1992) outlined above. Each narrative was analysed for use of story grammar and cohesive devices, as well as for developmental stage. Overall, the findings of Boon et al. (1994) showed that the ability of children treated for ALL to spontaneously generate a novel story was virtually the same as that of a group of age- and sex-matched, non-neurologically impaired control subjects. The narratives of the children treated for ALL did not differ to those collected from the control group on the majority of parameters assessed including: story length, number of episodes generated, proportion of complete episodes produced, frequency of use of story grammar categories, use of interepisodic relations, number of cohesive ties per proposition, use of cohesive categories, cohesive adequacy and developmental stage. The two groups did, however, differ significantly in the proportion of episodes containing Initiating Events, with the control group producing more episodes containing Initiating Events than the children treated for ALL.

Similar outcomes for spontaneously generated narratives have been reported by Jordan et al. (1991) for a group of children following closed head injury, and also by Hudson and Murdoch (1992) for a group of children with posterior fossa tumours (see above). In a study examining story recall abilities of normal and severely disabled readers, Weaver and Dickinson (1982) found that story grammar did not differentiate between the groups, and concluded that story grammars may be of limited diagnostic utility to distinguish between good and poor readers. It should be noted, however, that Mandler (1982) replied to this latter report by pointing out that one of the 'most interesting findings' from story grammar analyses has been the consistent patterns of recall of the various story grammar categories across a wide variety of populations and ages. Mandler (1982) concluded that such consistency suggests that the operation of a story schema may be a universal kind of functioning. Other subject groups have also been reported to demonstrate similar results to those reported by Weaver and Dickinson (1982). For instance, story grammar analysis has been reported to not differentiate between learning-disabled and normally achieving students (Graybeal, 1981; Weaver and Dickinson, 1982).

A number of studies exist in the developmental literature, however, which have found that children with developmental language deficits perform more poorly on a story grammar analysis than their age- and/or language-matched peers (Liles, 1985, 1987; Merritt and Liles, 1987; Olley, 1989). It may be that a distinction needs eventually to be drawn between developmental findings and acquired aetiologies. However, the limited amount of literature available restricts such a distinction being considered either advantageous or justifiable at present.

The only significant result recorded by Boon et al. (1994) was the measure of the number of episodes that contained Initiating Events. The control subjects produced significantly more episodes that contained Initiating Events than the ALL subjects. Thus, the ALL subjects tended to omit the beginnings of an episode, so the listener was more likely to be in ignorance of those events that caused the protagonist to act.

Although Roth and Spekman (1986) found that learning-disabled subjects produced significantly fewer episodes containing Responses, Attempts and Plans, when compared to their normally achieving peers, no difference was found with regard to the proportion of episodes containing Initiating Events. The finding of Boon et al. (1994) is similar to that of Weaver and Dickinson (1982) who, in a story recall study, found no difference between normal and disabled readers in the mean proportion of story grammar categories recalled.

Boon et al. (1994) reported no difference between the ALL and the control groups in the manner in which they linked episodes of their narratives. Of interest is the proportion of each relation used. In Stein and Glenn's (1979) study of three age groups — Kindergarten, Grade 3 and Grade 5 — a majority of the children's stories involved causal relations, with increasingly higher percentages appearing in the older two groups. In contrast, Boon et al. (1994) reported that both the ALL and the control groups evidenced a high proportion of 'Then' interepisodic relations, with the causal relations being used most infrequently out of the four interepisodic relations.

The length of the narrative generated by the children treated for ALL investigated by Boon et al. (1994) was not significantly different from that generated by their control subjects. This finding is in contrast to that of Roth and Spekman (1986), who found that, in a task involving the generation of a novel story, learning-disabled subjects produced stories that contained significantly fewer propositions (i.e. were shorter stories) than those produced by normally achieving peers.

The cohesion analysis carried out by Boon et al. (1994) did not reveal any significant differences in performance between the ALL and the control groups on the story generation task. The ALL subjects used the same average number of ties per proposition as the control subjects and demonstrated equally well-developed use of cohesive strategies, with no difference in the proportion of complete, incomplete and erroneous ties used. This finding is similar to that of Jordan et al. (1991), but contrasts with the findings of other researchers (Olley, 1989; Hudson and Murdoch, 1992), who reported that their impaired groups demonstrated fewer complete ties than the controls.

In summary, the findings of the study reported by Boon et al. (1994) indicated that the performance of children treated for ALL on a spontaneous narrative task was very similar to that of age- and sex-matched control subjects, both on story grammar and cohesive aspects. Since these same groups differed on normed structural measures of syntactic and semantic ability (see Chapter 6) this finding seems to question the claim that narrative analyses are sensitive to complex, integrated aspects of language functioning. It must be remembered, however, that narrative abilities constitute only one aspect of discourse, and there is, therefore, a need to examine other discourse abilities, such as conversation, before it can be concluded that the discourse abilities of ALL children are unimpaired. The same would be true for children treated for posterior fossa tumours. As yet, reports of the conversational abilities of children treated for neoplastic conditions have not appeared in the literature.

References

Applebee AN (1978) The Child's Concept of Story. Chicago, IL: University of Chicago Press.

Bloom L, Lahey M (1978) Language Development and Language Disorders. New York: John Wiley & Sons.

Boon DL, Murdoch BE, Jordan FM (1994) Performance on creative narrative tasks of children treated for acute lymphocytic leukaemia. Aphasiology 8: 549–568.

Botvin GJ, Sutton-Smith B (1977) The development of structural complexity in children's fantasy narratives. Developmental Psychology 14: 377–388.

Buttsworth DL, Murdoch BE, Ozanne AE (1983) Acute lymphoblastic leukaemia: language deficits in children post-treatment. Disability and Rehabilitation 15: 67–75.

Dennis M (1980) Strokes in childhood I: Communicative intent, expression, and comprehension after left hemisphere arteriopathy in a right-handed nine-year-old. In Rieber RW (ed.) Language Development and Aphasia in Children. New York: Academic Press: 45–67.

Ernest-Baron CR, Brookshire RH, Nicholas LE (1987) Story structure and retelling of narratives by aphasic and non-brain-damaged adults. Journal of Speech and Hearing Research 30: 44–49.

Graybeal CM (1981) Memory for stories in language-impaired children. Applied Psycholinguistics 3: 269–283.

Halliday MAK, Hasan R (1976) Cohesion in English. London: Longman Group.

Hartley LL (1986) Syntactic abilities of closed head injured patients in narrative discourse. Paper presented to the American Speech–Language–Hearing Association, Detroit, MI.

Hudson LJ, Murdoch BE (1992) Chronic language deficits in children treated for posterior fossa tumours. Aphasiology 6: 135–150.

Jackel CA, Murdoch BE, Ozanne AE, Buttsworth DL (1990) Language abilities of children treated for acute lymphoblastic leukaemia: preliminary findings. Aphasiology 4: 45–53.

Johnston JR (1982) Narratives: a new look at communication problems in older language-disordered children. Language, Speech and Hearing Services in Schools 13: 144–155.

Johnson NS, Mandler JM (1980) A tale of two structures: underlying and surface forms in stories. Poetics 9: 51–86.

Jordan FM, Murdoch BE, Buttsworth DL (1991) Closed-head-injured children's performance on narrative tasks. Journal of Speech and Hearing Research 34: 572–582.

Kemper S (1984) The development of narrative skills: explanation and entertainments. In Kuczaj SA (ed.) Discourse Development: Progress in Cognitive Development Research. New York: Springer-Verlag: 99–124.

Klecan-Aker JS, McIngvale GK, Swank PR (1987) Stimulus considerations in narrative analysis of normal third grade children. Language and Speech 30: 13–24.

Labov W (1972) Language in the Inner City: Studies in the Black English Vernacular. Philadelphia, PA: University of Pennsylvania.

Liles BZ (1985) Narrative ability in normal and language disordered children. Journal of Speech and Hearing Research 28: 123–133.

Liles BZ (1987) Episode organization and cohesive conjunctives in narratives of children with and without language disorders. Journal of Speech and Hearing Research 40: 185–196.

Mandler JM (1982) An analysis of story grammars. In Klix F, Hoffmann J, van der Meer E (eds) Cognitive Research in Psychology. Amsterdam: North Holland: 89–103.

Mandler JM, Johnson NS (1977) Remembrance of things parsed: story structure and recall. Cognitive Psychology 9: 111–151.

Merritt DD, Liles BZ (1987) Story grammar ability in children with and without language disorder: story generation, story retelling, and story comprehension. Journal of Speech and Hearing Research 30: 539–552.

Olley L (1989) Oral narrative performance of normal and language impaired school aged children. Australian Journal of Human Communication Disorders 17: 43–65.

Page JL, Stewart SR (1985) Story grammar skills in school-age children. Topics in Language Disorders March: 16–30.

Peterson C, McCabe A (1983) Developmental Psycholinguistics: Three Ways of Looking at a Child's Narrative. New York: Plenum Press.

Roth FP, Spekman NJ (1986) Narrative discourse: spontaneously generated stories of learning-disabled and normally achieving students. Journal of Speech and Hearing Disorders 51: 8–23.

Roth FP, Spekman NJ (1989) The oral syntactic proficiency of learning disabled students: a spontaneous story sampling analysis. Journal of Speech and Hearing Research 32: 67–77.

Rumelhart D (1975) Notes on a schema for stories. In Brown D, Collins A (eds) Representation and Understanding: Studies in Cognitive Science. New York: Academic Press: 211–236.

Stein NL, Glenn CG (1979) An analysis of story comprehension in school children. In Freedle RO (ed.) New Directions in Discourse Processing. New Jersey: Abelex Norwood: 53–120.

Swartzlander P, Naremore R (1989) Stories and scripts: performance of normal and language delayed preschoolers. Paper presented to the American Speech–Language–Hearing Association, St. Louis, MO.

Umiker-Sebeok DJ (1979) Preschool children's intraconversational narrative. Journal of Child Language 6: 91–109.

Weaver PA, Dickinson DK (1982) Scratching below the surface: exploring the usefulness of story grammars. Discourse Processes 5: 225–243.

Wiig EH, Semel E (1984) Language Assessment and Intervention for the Learning Disabled. Columbus, OH: Charles E Merrill.

Chapter 8
Motor speech disorders in children treated for brain tumours

BRUCE E MURDOCH, LISA J HUDSON AND
SUSAN K HORTON

Introduction

Brain tumours involving structures contained in the posterior cranial fossa account for more than half of all paediatric intracranial neoplasms (Naidich and Zimmerman, 1984; Segall et al., 1985) (see Chapter 1). In that mass lesions located in the posterior cranial fossa inevitably involve the cerebellum either directly or indirectly, it could be expected that features of ataxic dysarthria would dominate any resultant speech disorder. The major features of ataxic dysarthria identified by Darley et al. (1975) include: marked breakdown of articulation involving both consonants and vowels; the prosodic disorders of excess and equal stress, prolonged phonemes and prolonged intervals, dysrhythmia and monotony of pitch and loudness, occasionally broken by patterns of excess loudness variation, a generally slow rate; and some harshness of the voice. A number of authors have linked the presence of ataxic dysarthria in children with the presence of mass lesions in the posterior cranial fossa (Brown, 1985; Rekate et al., 1985; Volcan et al., 1986; Ammirati et al., 1989; Murdoch and Hudson-Tennent, 1994).

Rekate et al. (1985) reviewed six children between two and 11 years of age who had experienced acute bilateral damage to large areas of both cerebellar hemispheres as a consequence of posterior fossa tumour. Their sample included four children with medulloblastoma, one with astrocytoma and one with ependymoma. All six children were mute for one to three months following surgical removal of their tumours and were severely dysarthric during recovery. Unfortunately, only two of the six cases were described in any detail by Rekate and co-workers. One case, an eight-year-old girl, underwent total removal of a medulloblastoma, which was situated in the vermis. By three months post-surgery, her expressive language had fully recovered although a slow, monotonous speech pattern persisted. Two and a half years later, normal academic achievement and a mild residual cerebellar dysarthria were noted. A six-year-old boy with an astrocytoma involving the vermis and left cerebellar hemisphere was also described. He began speaking one month post-surgery, demonstrating 'characteristic cerebellar dysarthria', which made him difficult to understand. Six months later, his speech was described as normal.

Volcan et al. (1986) described another case of muteness immediately preceding dysarthria and subsequent to the removal of a posterior fossa tumour. They described an eight-year-old girl who had a medulloblastoma removed from the fourth ventricle, which resulted in a mild right paresis, truncal ataxia, signs of right cerebellar dysfunction, and muteness. Within two weeks she had regained monosyllabic speech but had a monotonous tone and was dysarthric. Vigorous work by her mother, a speech pathologist, preceded a marked improvement. Twelve months post-surgery, a mild dysarthria was still present.

Similarly, Ammirati et al. (1989) described the onset of mutism in a 14-year-old boy 24 hours after the complete excision of a vermian astrocytoma. Cranial nerve palsies, long tract signs, or dysphagia were, however, not detected. He was able to pronounce two-syllable words three weeks post-operatively and five weeks after surgery was dysarthric but able to produce two- and three-word utterances. At follow-up, four months post-surgery, he exhibited a mild residual dysarthria and minimal gait ataxia. The nature of the dysarthria observed was not described. Both Rekate et al. (1985) and Ammirati et al. (1989) postulated that the mutism observed in their cases may have been related to bilateral involvement of the dentate nuclei, and that the subsequent resolution of dysarthric speech may represent a recovering cerebellar mechanism.

With the exception of the study reported by Murdoch and Hudson-Tennent (1994) none of the studies listed above provide detailed descriptions of the dysarthrias observed in children following treatment for posterior fossa tumours. In addition, Murdoch and Hudson-Tennent (1994) appear to be the only authors to account for the presence or absence of developmental components in the observed speech disorders exhibited by these children. It must be recognized that as in other forms of acquired childhood dysarthria, many of the children treated for posterior fossa tumour are still developing speech at the time of central nervous system (CNS) trauma. Consequently, they cannot be expected to have consolidated adult skills in the areas of respiration, phonation, resonation or articulation and hence, their speech may be affected differently from that of adults. In that it represents the most comprehensive description of both the ataxic and developmental features of the dysarthrias exhibited by children following treatment for posterior fossa tumours reported to date, a synopsis of the study conducted by Murdoch and Hudson-Tennent (1994) follows.

Features of dysarthria following treatment for posterior fossa tumour

General features

Murdoch and Hudson-Tennent (1994) examined the speech production abilities of 19 children aged between 4;5 and 16;10 who had been treated for a posterior fossa tumour at least 12 months previously. Thirteen of the subjects had experienced a course of radiotherapy following surgical excision of their tumour and one subject had received both radiotherapy and chemotherapy post-surgery. The speech abilities of each child was assessed by way of two tests, which included the *Frenchay Dysarthria Assessment* (Enderby, 1983) and the *Fisher–Logemann Test of Articulation Competence* (Fisher and Logemann, 1971). In addition, a connected speech sample was obtained from each subject for the purpose of a perceptual analysis. The perceptual analysis involved each sample being rated by two independent judges on the 32 perceptual dimensions of speech originally described by Darley et al. (1975) and later modified by FitzGerald et al. (1987). These dimensions covered the five aspects of speech production: prosody (including features of pitch, loudness, rate, stress and phrasing), respiration, phonation, resonance and articulation. Overall intelligibility was also rated.

On the basis of the three different speech assessments, Murdoch and Hudson-Tennent (1994) determined that 11 of the 19 children treated for posterior fossa tumour were speech disordered. The performance of each of the 11 speech-disordered children on the three speech assessments is summarized in Table 8.1.

The deviant speech dimensions exhibited by the speech-disordered children are listed in descending order of frequency in Table 8.2.

The perceptual analysis showed that precision of consonants and nasality were the most commonly identified deviant speech dimensions exhibited by the speech-disordered children treated for posterior fossa tumour, with 72.7% of these children exhibiting an imprecise production of consonants and/or hyponasal (three children) or hypernasal (five children) speech. Reduced overall intelligibility followed, occurring in 63.6% of the children. Two of the 11 subjects exhibited a moderate reduction in speech intelligibility, whereas five demonstrated a just noticeable deviation in intelligibility. More than half of the speech-disordered children (54.5%) demonstrated a pitch level that was inappropriately high for their age and sex. Four children (36.4%) exhibited deviant stress patterns, strained–strangled vocal quality and a reduced general rate. In terms of the broad aspects of speech production rated, abnormalities of articulation and resonation were observed by Murdoch and Hudson-Tennent (1994) most frequently, followed by reduced overall intelligibility. The remaining deviant speech dimensions were predominantly those of prosody. Compared to a group of age- and sex-matched control subjects, Murdoch and Hudson-Tennent (1994) reported that overall intelligibility, precision of consonants and general stress were significantly more deviant in their speech-disordered children treated for posterior fossa tumour.

Murdoch and Hudson-Tennent (1994) reported that, based on their performance on the *Frenchay Dysarthria Assessment*, the speech-disordered children treated for posterior fossa tumour showed reduced abilities in the respiratory and laryngeal systems and in the functioning of the lips and tongue. Difficulties were indicated both at rest and during rapid speech and non-speech movements, suggesting involvement of abnormal muscle tone and of impaired co-ordination.

All but two of the 11 speech-disordered children examined by Murdoch and Hudson-Tennent (1994) demonstrated speech abnormalities when producing single words included in the *Fisher–Logemann Test of Articulation Competence* (see Table 8.1). Developmental errors, including phonological processes, articulatory substitutions and/or vowel distortions were present in the speech of eight of the 11 children treated for tumour. In seven of those eight subjects, these errors represented residual developmental errors that should have been eliminated from their speech. For example, residual developmental errors detected in the speech of tumour subject 8 (age 11;3) included among others, /f/ for /θ/ (medial position) and syllable reduction. The substitution /f/ for /θ/ usually resolves at the age of seven or eight years (Bernthal and Bankson, 1981) and syllable reduction usually disappears by four years of age (Grunwell, 1982). Subject 1, aged 4;5, was young enough not to warrant concern about the retention of some phonological processes (e.g. gliding, cluster reduction). In addition, Murdoch and Hudson-Tennent (1994) reported that the twin brother of Subject 1 exhibited similar phonological errors. Seven of the children treated for posterior fossa tumour exhibited articulatory substitutions, however, two of these demonstrated age-appropriate errors. Two of the speech-disordered children evidenced inconsistent articulatory errors and one child was reported by Murdoch and Hudson-Tennent (1994) to articulate all phonemes accurately but in a prolonged manner.

In summary, 11 (58%) of the 19 children treated for posterior fossa tumour examined by Murdoch and Hudson-Tennent (1994) exhibited acquired and/or developmental speech difficulties. Overall, the children identified as speech-disordered demonstrated mild dysarthric features as indicated by the reported predominance of 'just noticeable' severity ratings determined during the perceptual analysis (see Table 8.2). The generalization that dysarthric features are mild in the long term post-surgery is, however, tempered by the fact that a range of severity levels was reported to be present among the children treated for posterior fossa tumour.

Table 8.1 Summary of the deviant speech characteristics exhibited by the 11 speech-disordered children treated for posterior fossa tumour examined by Murdoch and Hudson-Tennent (1994)

Subject	Frenchay Dysarthria Assessment	Fisher–Logemann Test of Articulation Competence	Perceptual analysis
1	UA	Five phonological processes	Imprecise consonants Reduced intelligibility
2	Respiration at rest Lip movements Laryngeal time Tongue at rest Tongue movements	Five phonological processes Inconsistent errors Vowel distortions One articulatory substitution (age-appropriate)	Imprecise consonants Hypernasality Deviant prosody Reduced intelligibility
3	UA	Four phonological processes Articulatory substitutions (age-appropriate)	Imprecise consonants Deviant prosody Reduced intelligibility
4	Respiration at rest Lip movements Jaw movement Palate maintenance* Laryngeal time Pitch Volume Tongue at rest Tongue movements Intelligibility	Four phonological processes Articulatory substitutions (age-appropriate) Inconsistent errors	Imprecise consonants Hoarseness Hyponasality Deviant prosody Reduced intelligibility
5	Respiration at rest Volume Tongue at rest Tongue movements	Articulatory substitutions Vowel errors Inconsistent errors	Normal on all dimensions

Table 8.1 (contd)

Subject	Frenchay Dysarthria Assessment	Fisher–Logemann Test of Articulation Competence	Perceptual analysis
6	Respiration at rest Lip movements Laryngeal time Tongue at rest Tongue movements	Articulatory substitutions	Imprecise consonants Hypernasality Deviant prosody
7	Weak reflexes* Respiration* Lips* Jaw* Palate maintenance* Laryngeal function* Tongue* Intelligibility	Six phonological processes Articulatory substitutions	Imprecise consonants Harshness Strained–strangled Hypernasality Deviant prosody Reduced intelligibility
8	Respiration* Lip movements Palate in speech Pitch Volume Laryngeal function* Tongue* Intelligibility	Two phonological processes Articulatory substitutions	Imprecise consonants Hypernasality Reduced intelligibility
9	Respiration at rest Lip movements Pitch Volume Laryngeal function* Tongue movements Intelligibility	Accurate articulation for single words	Imprecise consonants Harshness Strained–strangled Hyponasality Deviant prosody

(contd)

Table 8.1 (contd)

Subject	Frenchay Dysarthria Assessment	Fisher–Logemann Test of Articulation Competence	Perceptual analysis
10	Respiration in speech Lips* Jaw* Palate maintenance Volume Laryngeal function Tongue Intelligibility	Accurate articulation for single words	Hoarseness Strained–strangled Hypernasality Deviant prosody
11	Respiration in speech Lips* Jaw in speech Palate maintenance* Pitch Volume Laryngeal function* Tongue* Intelligibility	Accurate articulation for single words but phonemes prolonged	Harshness Hoarseness Strained–strangled Hyponasality Deviant prosody Reduced intelligibility

* = All aspects of function impaired; UA = unavailable.

Table 8.2 Occurrence and severity of speech deviations found in the tumour group (N=11) examined by Murdoch and Hudson-Tennent (1994)

Speech deviation	Frequency of deviation in tumour sample		Severity of deviation					
			Just noticeable		Moderate		Severe	
	N	(%)	N	(%)	N	(%)	N	(%)
Precision of consonants	8	(72.7)	8	(100)	–	(–)	–	(–)
Nasality	8	(72.7)	7	(87.5)	1	(12.5)	–	(–)
Overall intelligibility	7	(63.6)	5	(71.4)	2	(28.6)	–	(–)
Pitch level	6	(54.5)	4	(66.7)	2	(33.3)	–	(–)
General stress	4	(36.4)	4	(100)	–	(–)	–	(–)
Strained–strangled	4	(36.4)	3	(75)	1	(25)	–	(–)
General rate	4	(36.4)	–	(–)	3	(75)	1	(25)
Hoarseness	3	(27.3)	2	(66.7)	1	(33.3)	–	(–)
Harshness	3	(27.3)	2	(66.7)	1	(33.3)	–	(–)
Prolonged intervals	3	(27.3)	3	(100)	–	(–)	–	(–)
Steadiness of pitch	2	(18.2)	2	(100)	–	(–)	–	(–)
Length of phonemes	2	(18.2)	2	(100)	–	(–)	–	(–)
Excessive loudness variation	2	(18.2)	2	(100)	–	(–)	–	(–)
Rate fluctuations	2	(18.2)	2	(100)	–	(–)	–	(–)
Maintenance of loudness	1	(9.1)	1	(100)	–	(–)	–	(–)
Mixed nasality	1	(9.1)	1	(100)	–	(–)	–	(–)
Pitch breaks	1	(9.1)	–	(–)	1	(100)	–	(–)
Excessive pitch fluctuations	1	(9.1)	1	(100)	–	(–)	–	(–)

Ataxic features

The earliest description of dysarthria associated with cerebellar disease was provided by Darley et al. (1969). In their study of 30 adult patients with cerebellar disease, Darley and co-workers determined imprecise consonants and excess and equal stress to be the most prominent deviant characteristics. In fact, the dimension of excess and equal stress was found to be more deviant in the group of patients with a cerebellar lesion than in any other aetiological group. Irregular articulatory breakdown was the third most prominent feature identified in the subject group of Darley et al. (1969). This feature was not specifically rated by the scale used by Murdoch and Hudson-Tennent (1994), however, inconsistent articulatory errors were noted by these authors in three of their children treated for posterior fossa tumour during completion of the *Fisher–Logemann Test of Articulation Competence*. The three speech dimensions reported by Murdoch and Hudson-Tennent (1994) to best differentiate their children treated for brain tumours from control subjects were precision of consonants, overall intelligibility and general stress. Although these represent very general dysarthric features, common to several different dysarthria types, they have also been identified as the most prominent characteristics of speech disorders associated with cerebellar damage (Darley et al, 1969; Kent and Netsell, 1975; Kent et al., 1979; Chenery et al., 1990).

In addition to the speech dimensions of prosodic excess and articulatory inaccuracy identified by Darley et al. (1975), a cluster of deviant speech dimensions entitled, phonatory prosodic insufficiency, was found to be prominent in patients with cerebellar lesions. Examination of the frequency table of deviant speech dimensions (Table 8.2) shows that 13 of the 18 dysarthric features demonstrated by the children treated for posterior fossa tumours examined by Murdoch and Hudson-Tennent (1994) could be classified as either phonatory or prosodic deviations (i.e. all features demonstrated with the exception of precision of consonants, nasality, mixed nasality, overall intelligibility and length of phonemes).

Following the work of Darley et al. (1975), a number of researchers have attempted to quantify objectively the perceived speech characteristics of ataxic dysarthria. For example, Kent and Netsell (1975) applied cineradiographic and spectrographic techniques to the speech of a single ataxic subject and confirmed the presence and nature of the deviant cluster entitled articulatory inaccuracy. Their subject evidenced reduced tongue movements in the anterior–posterior dimension, distorted vowel productions and consonant articulations that were either incorrect or omitted entirely. Murdoch and Hudson-Tennent (1994) reported imprecision of consonant production to be a significant deviant speech dimension in their group of speech-disordered children treated for posterior fossa tumours.

The prominence of excess and equal stress in the speech of subjects with cerebellar disease was confirmed by Kent et al. (1979) using acoustic analyses to detect the lengthening of phonemes that are normally brief in duration. Consequently, the range of syllable durations utilized by normal speakers is significantly reduced in speakers with cerebellar disease, resulting in the perception that excess and equal stress is being placed on usually unstressed speech segments. The findings of Murdoch and Hudson-Tennent (1994) indicate that this distinctive feature of dysarthria associated with cerebellar disease is apparent not only in the speech of adults but also in children with cerebellar lesions.

Quantifiable evidence of the cluster, phonatory prosodic insufficiency, was established by Kent and Rosenbek (1982). Spectrographic analyses revealed the presence of a flat fundamental frequency associated with ataxic dysarthria, as well as the production of consecutive syllables without variation in the intonation pattern. Monopitch and monoloudness were not identified in the speech-disordered children treated for posterior fossa tumours studied by Murdoch and Hudson-Tennent (1994). Instead, they reported that large fluctuations in pitch and loudness were demonstrated by their tumour subjects as indicated by the judges' perception of the deviant dimensions: steadiness of pitch, excessive loudness variation, maintenance of loudness, pitch breaks and excessive fluctuation of pitch. Impaired control of fundamental frequency was objectively established as a prominent characteristic in the ataxic subject studied by Kent and Netsell (1975).

Chenery et al. (1990) analysed the speech of 16 adults with a diagnosed cerebellar disorder using the same series of 32 speech dimensions employed by Murdoch and Hudson-Tennent (1994). The most frequent deviant speech dimension identified by Chenery et al. (1990) was that of general stress pattern. This was followed closely by deficits in consonant precision, pitch variation, general rate of speech, length of intervals and a harsh vocal quality. When compared to a control group, the ataxic subjects were significantly less intelligible and scored significantly below the control group on many speech dimensions, including precision of consonants and general stress patterns. The ataxic adults studied by Chenery et al. (1990) appeared to demonstrate dysarthric features, which were of a greater degree of severity than those exhibited by the children examined by Murdoch and Hudson-Tennent (1994). The deviant features of overall intelligibility, general stress pattern and precision of consonants, however, were prominent in both groups, further supporting the hypothesis that children treated for posterior fossa tumour are likely to have residual ataxic features in their speech.

Murdoch and Hudson-Tennent (1994) utilized the *Frenchay Dysarthria Assessment* to evaluate the oromotor skills of their tumour subjects. Included in the manual of the *Frenchay Dysarthria Assessment* is a performance profile obtained by adult subjects with cerebellar lesions. When this was compared to the profile obtained by the children treated for posterior fossa tumour included in Murdoch and Hudson-Tennent's (1994) study, many similarities were evident. The areas in which reduced abilities were most evident in the children treated for posterior fossa tumours included respiration, lips, larynx and tongue. These features were also impaired in the adult subjects studied by Enderby (1983), however, Enderby determined a marked difference between the subjects' intact oromotor functioning at rest and their poorly co-ordinated abilities during speech or non-speech movements. Overall, the speech-disordered children investigated by Murdoch and Hudson-Tennent (1994) exhibited a reduction in respiratory, lip, laryngeal and tongue function both at rest and during movement, suggesting that both flaccid and ataxic components are present in the observed speech disorder. The flaccidity may be attributed to the cranial nerve damage diagnosed in three subjects immediately post-surgery. Examination of the remaining 16 subjects' *Frenchay Dysarthria Assessment* profiles did not reveal the presence of flaccid oromuscular functioning suggesting that the primary effects of posterior fossa tumour were ataxic in nature.

Developmental features

The major variable which differentiates adult and paediatric dysarthric subjects is the co-occurrence of developmental errors and dysarthric features in many children who suffer an acquired brain lesion. Murdoch and Hudson-Tennent (1994) reported that the *Fisher–Logemann Test of Articulation Competence* revealed the presence of developmental errors in eight of the 11 speech-disordered subjects included in their study. Seven of the eight subjects were reported to be using phonological processes, articulatory substitution, and/or vowel distortions, which should have already been eliminated from their speech. The remaining subject (Subject 1), aged 4;5 at assessment, had retained the same phonological processes as his twin brother, thus complicating any assumptions that could be made about the nature of his speech disorder.

It is of note that all eight children exhibiting developmental speech errors investigated by Murdoch and Hudson-Tennent (1994) were aged less than six years at the time of tumour diagnosis and treatment (range 1;9–5;9). The three subjects who demonstrated mature speech sound systems were aged from 10;6 to 12;0 at the time of tumour onset and, hence, had already acquired and consolidated all of the speech sounds and phonological rules of English. Also worthy of mention is the fact that the eight children treated for posterior fossa tumour who performed normally on all three assessment measures were older than six years of age at the time of CNS trauma (range 6;1–13;3).

It would appear that CNS trauma sustained during the early developing years has the potential to interrupt normal speech development and introduce dysarthric features to speech and non-speech functions. The characteristics of dysarthria identified in the children treated for posterior fossa tumour by Murdoch and Hudson-Tennent (1994) can be attributed to the posterior fossa site of the tumours and their surgical removal. The impact of posterior fossa tumours and their treatment on speech development is less clear. It is possible that the cerebellum has a role in the learning of new motor programmes (Sanes et al., 1990). Whilst the influence of cerebellar lesions on the execution of motor programmes has frequently been addressed (e.g. Darley et al., 1969; Chenery et al., 1990), the potential for cerebellar damage to impair the acquisition of new motor skills has only recently been considered.

For example, Sanes et al. (1990) evaluated the improvement exhibited by 11 adults with cerebellar atrophy when repeatedly tracing an irregular geometric pattern. The observation that any improvements in speed were offset by reductions in accuracy suggested to Sanes et al. (1990) that the subject group did not demonstrate motor skill learning. It was considered that the subjects were merely altering their performance strategy in an attempt to cope with the task. Sanes et al. (1990) concluded that the cerebellum and its associated pathways are critical in the motor learning process. Should such theories of cerebellar functioning apply to the acquisition of motor speech skills, then difficulties may be anticipated when children treated for posterior fossa tumour attempt to learn mature motor speech skills. Cerebellar involvement may prevent their progression through the developmental continuum to an adult standard of speech.

Factors contributing to motor speech impairment following treatment for posterior fossa tumours

In discussing the nature and severity of speech disorders occurring subsequent to the treatment of posterior fossa tumour, the variables which are unique to this aetiology must also be considered. Firstly, the majority of tumour types experienced by the children included in the study conducted by Murdoch and Hudson-Tennent (1994) do not infiltrate the cerebellar structures but exert pressure on the cerebellum. Consequently, provided surgical excision can be performed without direct damage occurring to any neural structures, a favourable prognosis may be anticipated. In three of the cases reported by Murdoch and Hudson-Tennent (1994), damage incurred during surgery contributed a flaccid component to the observed ataxic and developmental speech disorders.

Secondly, nine of the 11 speech-disordered children reported by Murdoch and Hudson-Tennent (1994) received a course of craniospinal irradiation post-surgery. The potential for radiotherapy to cause long-term CNS damage, particularly to young children, has been reviewed elsewhere (see Hudson et al., 1990). The effects of radiotherapy may negatively influence the prognosis for speech abilities and may interrupt normal speech development. In other words, the dysarthric and developmental features observed by Murdoch and Hudson-Tennent (1994) may not be a direct result of cerebellar damage subsequent to tumour or surgery, but may be secondary to damage caused by CNS irradiation.

A third characteristic, which has been observed in some children treated for posterior fossa tumour is the occurrence of muteness post-surgery. A number of authors have described children who were mute immediately or soon after surgical excision of posterior fossa tumours (Rekate et al., 1985; Volcan et al., 1986; Ammirati et al., 1989). Previous studies have described children who were mute from two weeks to three months and were severely dysarthric when their speech returned. A mild residual dysarthria was likely to persist in the long term. Unfortunately, descriptive details of the reported dysarthrias were not provided by these authors. Four of the children treated for posterior fossa tumours examined by Murdoch and Hudson-Tennent (1994) were reportedly mute post-surgery and dysarthric during the recovery period. However, these authors also noted that many of their subjects exhibited dysarthric features without having experienced muteness post-surgery. This finding suggests that while the occurrence of muteness following the surgical removal of a posterior fossa tumour is a precursor of dysarthria, the absence of muteness post-surgery does not allow the prediction of intact speech abilities in the long term.

Overall, the findings of Murdoch and Hudson-Tennent (1994) serve to demonstrate that while disorders of speech are not an inevitable consequence of posterior fossa tumour treatment in children, both developmental and acquired speech characteristics can occur. Further, it would appear that many of the ataxic features previously documented in adult subjects with cerebellar lesions may also be experienced by children with cerebellar involvement. As noted by Murdoch and Hudson-Tennent (1994), however, the speech difficulties observed in children treated for posterior fossa tumours are further complicated by the interaction between the acquired and developmental components of the disorder.

Physiological assessment of dysarthria following treatment for posterior fossa tumours

As outlined above, Murdoch and Hudson-Tennent (1994) used a range of perceptual assessments of dysarthria to describe the motor speech disorders exhibited by children treated for posterior fossa tumours. Although perceptual assessments of dysarthria are clinically significant and helpful for diagnostic purposes (Hirose, 1986), they have a number of inherent inadequacies that limit their usefulness in determining treatment priorities (Ludlow and Bassich, 1983). It is now widely acknowledged that an understanding of the underlying pathophysiology of the speech production mechanism, determined by way of physiological, instrumental measures, is necessary for the development of optimal treatments for motor speech disorders (Abbs and DePaul, 1989). To date, however, physiological investigations of the functioning of the speech production mechanism in children with dysarthria subsequent to acquired damage to the CNS have been rarely reported (Bak et al., 1983; Murdoch and Hudson-Tennent, 1993; van Dongen et al., 1994). The case described below presents a comprehensive perceptual and physiological profile of the function of the major motor subsystems of the speech production mechanism of a child treated for posterior fossa tumour. In particular, the results of the physiological assessments carried out in this case demonstrate the potential importance of physiological instruments in defining treatment priorities for children with acquired dysarthria. Further details of the perceptual and physiological measures used to assess the case reported below are provided in Chapter 9.

Case report

Rebecca was an 8-year-old, right-handed female who had been admitted to hospital at 6 years of age with severe ataxia. A magnetic resonance imaging scan soon after admission revealed the presence of a large cerebellar astrocytoma (see Figure 8.1). The tumour was subsequently removed surgically. During the operation, the left cerebellar hemisphere was completely removed, along with a large portion of the right cerebellar hemisphere. Neither radiotherapy nor chemotherapy were administered as part of the treatment regimen.

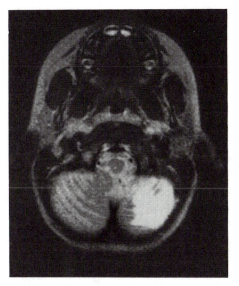

Figure 8.1 Rebecca: MRI scan showing a large astrocytoma in the posterior cranial fossa

Rebecca was administered a comprehensive battery of perceptual and physiological dysarthria assessments at approximately 2 years post-surgery, at which time she was mildly dysarthric.

The perceptual assessments administered to Rebecca included: the *Assessment of Intelligibility of Dysarthric Speech* (Yorkston and Beukelman, 1981), which provides an index of severity of dysarthric speech by quantifying both single-word and sentence intelligibility, as well as speaking rate of dysarthric speakers; the *Frenchay Dysarthria Assessment* (Enderby, 1983), which provides a standardized assessment of speech neuromuscular activity; and a perceptual analysis of a speech sample (FitzGerald et al., 1987) based on a rating scale involving 32 deviant speech dimensions encompassing prosody, respiration, phonation, resonance and articulation.

Rebecca's respiratory, laryngeal, velopharyngeal and articulatory function was also assessed instrumentally using a battery of specialized, physiological instruments. Respiratory function was assessed, using both spirometric and kinematic techniques as described by Murdoch and Hudson-Tennent (1993) and included measures such as vital capacity, forced expiratory volume per second, percentage of relative contribution of the rib cage, lung volume initiation and termination levels during production of a range of speech tasks, mean syllables per breath, speaking rate and the incidence of slope changes and paradoxical chest wall movements. One other indicator of respiratory function for speech, namely sub-glottal pressure, was estimated by use of an Aerophone II (Kay Elemetrics) airflow measurement system consistent with the method described by Theodoros and Murdoch (1994).

Vocal fold vibration and laryngeal aerodynamics were assessed using electroglottography and an airflow measurement system (Aerophone II), respectively. The parameters measured in these assessments included fundamental frequency (Fo), duty cycle, closing time, ab/adduction rate, sound pressure level, glottal resistance and phonatory flow rate. Velopharyngeal function was assessed using the accelerometric technique described by Theodoros et al. (1993), which provides a nasality index (the Horii Oral Nasal Coupling Index). The assessment of articulatory function involved measurement of lip and tongue strength, endurance and rate of repetitive movements using strain-gauge and pressure transduction systems. The transducer used for assessing tongue function was identical to the rubber-bulb pressure transducer described by Murdoch et al. (1995). A miniaturized pressure transducer, based on semiconductor strain-gauge technology similar to that described by Hinton and Luschei (1992), was used to estimate lip strength and endurance. In addition, changes in the dimensions of the lips during performance of speech and non-speech tasks were monitored by a quantifiable video assessment procedure.

The perceptual assessments indicated that Rebecca had a mild dysarthria, characterized primarily by a slow rate of speech and an equal and even stress pattern. Some impairment in articulation was noted, with lip function being mildly affected and tongue function moderately impaired. On the basis of the perceptual assessments there was no evidence of impairments in the processes of respiration, phonation or velopharyngeal function. Intelligibility was found to be only mildly affected.

In contrast to the perceptual findings, however, instrumental analysis revealed that Rebecca had below normal lung volumes and capacities. In addition, she was primarily an abdominal breather and demonstrated an overall reduction in chest wall excursion during performance of a range of different speech tasks. Instrumental investigation of laryngeal and velopharyngeal function confirmed that these subsystems were performing within normal limits. As suggested by the perceptual assessments, some evidence of articulatory dysfunction was detected by the strain-gauge and pressure transducers. Maximum lip pressure on non-speech tasks was reduced as were the lip pressures achieved by Rebecca when producing bilabial consonants. However, this did not lead to a noticeable distortion of bilabial consonants. Tongue pressure and endurance levels were within normal limits although Rebecca's repetitive tongue movements were slow. It is suggested that in the latter task, Rebecca reduced the number of repetitions to preserve the strength and accuracy of her tongue movements.

In summary, subsequent to surgical removal of her posterior fossa tumour, Rebecca presented with a mild dysarthria characterized primarily by prosodic disorders including a slow rate of speech and poor intonation. The physiological assessments also revealed some respiratory and articulatory problems, which may well contribute to the prosodic disorder. For instance, it is possible that Rebecca may have reduced her rate of speech in order to conserve expiratory output and to ensure accuracy and strength of articulatory movements. Importantly, the physiological analysis was able to identify dysfunction at some levels of the speech production mechanism not evidenced by the perceptual assessments, thereby highlighting the advantage of instrumental analysis over perceptual assessments in defining treatment goals for children with acquired dysarthria. It is recommended that when designing programmes for the treatment of dysarthria occurring in children subsequent to treatment for posterior fossa tumours, clinicians base their decisions on a combination of both perceptual and physiological measures.

References

Abbs J, De Paul R (1989) Assessment of dysarthria: the critical prerequisite to treatment. In Leahy MM (ed.) Disorders of Communication: The Science of Intervention. London: Taylor & Francis: 206–227.

Ammirati M, Mirzai S, Samii M (1989) Transient mutism following removal of a cerebellar tumour: a case report and review of the literature. Child's Nervous System 5: 12–14.

Bak E, Van Dongen HR, Arts WFM (1983) The analysis of acquired dysarthria in childhood. Developmental Medicine and Child Neurology 25: 81–94.

Bernthal JE, Bankson NW (1981) Articulation Disorders. Englewood Cliffs, NJ: Prentice-Hall.

Brown JK (1985) Dysarthria in children: neurologic perspective. In Darby JK (ed.) Speech and Language Evaluaton in Neurology: Childhood Disorders. Orlando, FL: Grune & Stratton: 133–184.

Chenery HJ, Ingram J, Murdoch BE (1990) Perceptual analysis of the speech in ataxic dysarthria. Australian Journal of Communication Disorders 18: 19–28.

Darley FL, Aronson AE, Brown JR (1969) Differential diagnostic patterns of dysarthria. Journal of Speech and Hearing Research 12: 246–269.

Darley FL, Aronson AE, Brown JR (1975) Motor Speech Disorders. Philadelphia, PA: WB Saunders.

Enderby P (1983) Frenchay Dysarthria Assessment. San Diego, CA: College-Hill Press.

Fisher HB, Logemann JA (1971) The Fisher–Logemann Test of Articulation Competence. Boston, MA: Houghton Mifflin.

FitzGerald FJ, Murdoch BE, Chenery HJ (1987) Multiple sclerosis: associated speech and language disorders. Australian Journal of Communication Disorders 15: 15–35.

Grunwell P (1982) Clinical Phonology. London: Croom Helm.

Hinton VA, Luschei ES (1992) Validation of a modern miniature transducer for measurement of interlabial contact pressure during speech. Journal of Speech and Hearing Research 35: 245–251.

Hirose H (1986) Pathophysiology of motor speech disorders (dysarthria). Folia Phoniatrica 38: 61–88.

Hudson LJ, Buttsworth DL, Murdoch BE (1990) Effect of CNS prophylaxis on speech and language function in children. In Murdoch BE (ed.) Acquired Neurological Speech/Language Disorders in Childhood. London: Taylor & Francis: 269–307.

Kent R, Netsell R (1975) A case study of an ataxic dysarthric: cineradiographic and spectrographic observations. Journal of Speech and Hearing Disorders 40: 115–134.

Kent RD, Rosenbek JC (1982) Prosodic disturbance and neurologic lesion. Brain and Language 15: 259–291.

Kent RD, Netsell R, Abbs JH (1979) Acoustic characteristics of dysarthria associated with cerebellar disease. Journal of Speech and Hearing Research 22: 627–648.

Ludlow CL, Bassich CJ (1983) The results of acoustic and perceptual assessment of two types of dysarthria. In Berry WR (ed.) Clinical Dysarthria. San Diego, CA: College-Hill Press: 121–154.

Murdoch BE, Hudson-Tennent LJ (1993) Speech breathing anomalies in children with dysarthria following treatment for posterior fossa tumours. Journal of Medical Speech–Language Pathology 1: 107–119.

Murdoch BE, Hudson-Tennent LJ (1994) Speech disorders in children treated for posterior fossa tumours: ataxic and developmental features. European Journal of Disorders of Communication 29: 379–397.

Murdoch BE, Attard M, Ozanne AE (1995) Impaired tongue strength and endurance in developmental verbal dyspraxia: a physiological analysis. European Journal of Communication Disorders 30: 51–64.

Naidich TP, Zimmerman RA (1984) Primary brain tumours in children. Seminars in Roentgenology 19: 100–114.

Rekate HL, Grubb RL, Aram DM, Hahn JF, Ratcheson RA (1985) Muteness of cerebellar origin. Archives of Neurology 42: 697–698.

Sanes JN, Dimitrov B, Hallett M (1990) Motor learning in patients with cerebellar dysfunction. Brain 113: 103–120.

Segall HD, Batnitzky S, Zee S, Ahmadi J, Bird CR, Cohen ME (1985) Computed tomography in the diagnosis of intracranial neoplasms in children. Cancer 56: 1748–1755.

Theodoros DG, Murdoch BE (1994) Laryngeal dysfunction in dysarthric speakers following severe closed head injury. Brain Injury 8: 667–684.

Theodoros DG, Murdoch BE, Stokes PD (1993) Hypernasality in dysarthric speakers following severe closed head injury: a perceptual and instrumental analysis. Brain Injury 7: 59–69.

van Dongen HR, Catsman-Berrevoets CE, Van Mourik M (1994) The syndrome of cerebellar mutism and subsequent dysarthria. Neurology 44: 2040–2046.

Volcan I, Cole GP, Johnston K (1986) A case of muteness of cerebellar origin [Letter to the Editor]. Archives of Neurology 43: 313–314.

Yorkston J, Beukelman D (1981) Assessment of Intelligibility of Dysarthric Speech. Austin, TX: Pro-Ed.

Chapter 9
Assessment and treatment of speech and language disorders occurring subsequent to cancer therapy in children

SUSAN K HORTON AND BRUCE E MURDOCH

Introduction

Each child surviving cancer has a unique history and combination of possible sequelae, including speech, language and cognitive deficits. The situation for the ever-increasing percentage of survivors of childhood cancer is that, although they may not have an ongoing chronic neoplastic disorder, they may have other complications (e.g. physical, social or psychological complications) resulting from the treatment applied to their cancer, which may continue indefinitely. This impairment in the status of the child, has been defined as the inability to participate fully in developmentally appropriate activities (Pantell and Lewis, 1987) and may manifest itself by a lack of adequate physical, emotional, or intellectual development (Jenney et al., 1995). This poses a challenge for healthcare professionals in their consideration of the need for follow-up services for this population. Evidence regarding the speech and language skills of the childhood cancer survivor, although indicating that dysarthria and language impairment are not inevitable outcomes (Hudson et al., 1989; Murdoch and Ozanne, 1993; Buttsworth et al., 1993), points to the need for long-term monitoring of these skills based on thorough and ongoing assessment. This assessment and monitoring may then indicate the need for individualized treatment of communication deficits if they are identified or as they arise.

Overview of speech and language disorders subsequent to cancer therapy in childhood

A clear reporting of the possible speech and language deficits occurring subsequent to cancer therapy in childhood is clouded by several factors,

187

including the nature of previous studies, the individual variation in subjects, the age at onset of the disease, the different cancer treatment regimens applied and the long-term sequelae of cancer treatments. As outlined earlier (see Chapters 3, 4, 5, 6 and 8) there are reports throughout the literature of communication disturbances in some children following therapy for various forms of childhood cancer (Broadbent et al., 1981; Danoff et al., 1982; Koh et al., 1994). Unfortunately, many of these studies do not offer specific descriptions of the nature of the communicative disturbances, and report cases and data in variable ways that prevent comparison. The reports are often based on reviews of hospital charts or retrospective reporting from medical professionals or parents (Carrow-Woolfolk and Lynch, 1982). A further complication to gaining a clear understanding of the nature of these communication disturbances is the wide variation in speech and language impairments observed from case to case as reported by Murdoch and Hudson-Tennent (1994) (see Chapter 5) and Murdoch et al. (1994) (see Chapter 6). This variation may have been hidden in some studies by the necessity of quantitative analysis of group data for statistical purposes, rather than pursuing the qualitative examination of data on an individual basis, the latter being more useful to the clinician for determining treatment priorities. As demonstrated by Murdoch and Hudson-Tennent (1994) and Murdoch et al. (1994), examination of each survivor of childhood cancer on a case-by-case basis is necessary to identify the significant individual differences in speech and language outcome that are essential for planning treatment for each subject's speech and language deficits.

Further, Paul (1995) reported that the long-term sequelae of therapy for childhood cancer can be subtle and variable depending on the timing of the therapy, as well as the location, size and area of the brain damaged by the treatments applied. Severity can range from almost non-existent to severe accompanying cognitive disturbances. A further complication of treatment for childhood cancer is the finding that language deficits in particular may not appear during routine communication tasks, but may surface during complex tasks such as those required at school (i.e. higher-level language, literacy and problem- solving skills). Indeed, the negative effects of radiotherapy have been reported to appear as delayed reactions, so that any associated language or cognitive deficit may only appear in the long term (Hudson et al., 1989). Nevertheless, there is considerable evidence that specific speech and language deficits may be expected in children following cancer therapy (see Chapters 3 and 6).

Speech disorders

Cerebellar or ataxic dysarthria is a frequently reported sequelae of the excision of posterior fossa tumours in childhood (Rekate et al., 1985; Murdoch and Hudson-Tennent, 1994). Other speech disorders have also been reported, including mixed ataxic-flaccid dysarthria (Hudson et al., 1989). The key features of these dysarthrias include imprecise consonants, hyper- or hypo-nasality, overall reduction in intelligibility and problems with pitch and stress. Transient mutism has been reported as a precursor to ataxic dysarthria in some children following the surgical removal of posterior fossa tumours (Rekate et al., 1985; Volcan et al., 1986; Hudson et al., 1989). This mutism has been reported to last for variable periods of time and must be considered to be part of a child's communication disorder following cancer therapy.

Murdoch and Hudson-Tennent (1994) caution clinicians to look further than dysarthria when examining the speech disorders following neurological damage in childhood by demonstrating the co-existence of dysarthria with developmental articulatory and phonological features in some of their child subjects. They emphasized the need to consider the developmental status of the child's speech at the time of the cancer therapy. Murdoch and Hudson-Tennent (1994) found developmental speech errors in the children who were less than six years of age at the time of tumour diagnosis and treatment. Children of this age have not completely acquired and consolidated all of the speech sounds and phonological rules of English. Further to this the authors postulated a likely interaction between central nervous system (CNS) damage and subsequent dysarthria on the developmental progression of a child's speech and conversely the possibility of developmental speech patterns having an effect on a listener's perception of dysarthric features.

In summary, following treatment for cancer, a child may present with a motor speech disorder in the form of dysarthria with or without developmental articulatory and phonological features. The nature of the speech disorder is largely dependent on the timing and nature of the cancer and its treatment and the developmental status of the child's speech prior to this.

Language disorders

The findings with regard to the language impairment following treatment for childhood cancer are much less clear-cut than for speech. Early reports tended to emphasize the relative sparing of children's language skills following treatment for childhood cancer (Eiser, 1978, 1980; Copeland et al., 1985). However, in these studies, effects on language may have been missed owing to the lack of sufficiently sensitive or specifically designed measures of language (Buttsworth et al., 1993). With advances in assessment techniques and more targeted investigations it is now accepted that language skills are often affected (see Chapters 3 and 6) and that the effects may be delayed or progressive due to the effects of radio- and chemotherapy on the CNS and therefore on language development in its later stages. This is even more significant as it is now accepted that language development and particularly the learning of discourse skills continues throughout childhood and the school-age years and into adolescence (Johnston, 1982).

Cognition

A final facet of the consideration of language impairment in children following treatment for childhood cancer is the interplay between cognition and language skills. Garcia-Perez et al. (1994) investigated the effects of brain irradiation, surgery and chemotherapy on the neuropsychological skills of children. They found a significant decline in the full-scale intelligence quotient from pre-illness to post-treatment for a population of children who suffered from intra-cranial tumours. Differences occurred in both performance (e.g. picture completion, picture arrangement subtests) and language-based skills (e.g. verbal fluency, verbal and visual memory). The researchers found in particular that children who underwent brain irradiation deteriorated in a number of specific cognitive functions. The most affected function was memory, followed by attention capacity, verbal fluency and sequential processing. All of these are key factors in the development and maintenance of good communication skills.

Buttsworth et al. (1993) reviewed reports on the possible intellectual impairment of children diagnosed with, and treated for, acute lymphoblastic leukaemia (ALL). The reports reviewed found subtle but significant lowering of intelligence quotients in long-term survivors of ALL. It was found that verbal associate reasoning and reasoning with abstract material were particularly vulnerable to interference from the effects of treatment for ALL.

Cognitive impairment must therefore be considered in concert with language impairment in children following treatment for cancer.

Assessment of the speech and language skills of children following cancer therapy

Early detection of any speech and language disorder following treatment for childhood cancer must be a priority for speech/language clinicians. Further to this, Buttsworth et al. (1993) believe that ongoing monitoring of skills must be maintained due to the possibility of language impairment as a late effect of treatment.

Assessment of speech

In order for treatment to be specific and targeted to the needs of the individual client, it must be driven by thorough and valid assessment. Speech assessment must take into account the possible developmental nature of some of the speech deficits, particularly if the child was younger than six years of age at the time of cancer detection and therapy.

A comprehensive assessment battery based on perceptual and physiological measures must be used if the presence of dysarthria is suspected. For a full discussion of the issues involved and the assessment instruments used in the assessment of children with dysarthria see Murdoch and Horton (1998).

Perceptual assessment

The section below outlines a recommended perceptual assessment battery that has been used by the authors for several years to assess the speech abilities of children treated for cancer. The same battery was used to assess the child presented in the case study at the end of this chapter. An articulation test such as the *Fisher–Logemann Test of Articulation Competence* (Fisher and Logemann, 1971) is included to provide an articulation profile as well as a simple phonological analysis by transcribing each target word in full, rather than just noting the target phonemes. This procedure aids in detecting and documenting the presence of developmental errors. The *Frenchay Dysarthria Assessment* (Enderby, 1983) is also included to provide a standardized assessment of speech neuromuscular activity, including respiration, articulation, resonance, phonation and speech-related reflex activity. Although designed for the adult population, this tool is suitable for use with children.

The *Assessment of Intelligibility of Dysarthric Speakers* (Yorkston and Beukelman, 1981) provides an index of severity of dysarthric speech by quantifying both single-word and sentence intelligibility as well as the speaking rate of dysarthric speakers. The final component in the recommended perceptual assessment battery for children with dysarthria is a perceptual analysis of a speech sample. The speech sample can be based on the child reading a standard passage such as 'The Grandfather Passage' (Darley et al., 1975) or, if the child cannot read, a picture description task. The sample is then rated by two judges, both qualified, experienced speech pathologists, on a series of 32 deviant dimensions of speech, originally described by Darley et al. (1975) and modified by FitzGerald et al., (1987). The dimensions pertain to the five aspects of speech production: prosody (including features of pitch, loudness, rate, stress and phrasing), respiration, phonation, resonance and articulation and overall intelligibility of speech.

Physiological assessment

The aim of physiological assessment of the speech mechanism is to compliment and extend the information obtained through perceptual assessment. It is an objective way of determining the severity and physiological nature of malfunctions of the speech mechanism. To be of value in deciding treatment priorities, the physiological assessment should be comprehensive, covering as many components of the speech production apparatus as possible. For a full discussion of the use of physiological assessment with children, the reader is directed to Murdoch and Horton (1998). The physiological assessment battery outlined below was used by the authors to assess the case reported in Chapter 8 and at the end of this chapter. The physiological assessment battery presented covers all four speech subsystems, these are, the respiratory, laryngeal, velopharyngeal and articulatory subsystems.

Evaluation of respiration

A spirometric assessment of respiratory function is used to estimate standard lung volumes and capacities. Values are compared to predicted values taking into account the subject's age, sex and height using the formulae provided by Boren et al. (1966) and Kory et al. (1961). Recording of the performance of the respiratory system during speech production is carried out using either the computerized strain-gauge belt pneumograph system developed by Murdoch et al. (1989) or inductance plethysmography (Respitrace). Briefly, these systems involve simultaneous, but independent, recording of circumferential size changes of the rib cage and abdomen. The rib cage and abdominal components of the respiratory system must be co-ordinated in their respective movements in that they each contribute simultaneously to changes in total lung volume and the production of sub-glottal air pressures during speech. Knowledge of how lung volume changes are partitioned between the various components of the respiratory apparatus (i.e. the rib cage and abdomen) is, therefore, of fundamental importance to understanding the physiological bases of both normal and disordered speech production.

One other important indicator of respiratory function for speech production is the ability of the subject to generate sub-glottal air pressure during speech (Netsell et al., 1989). Sub-glottal air pressure can be estimated using the Aerophone II (Kay Elemetrics) airflow measurement system.

Evaluation of laryngeal function

Physiological evaluation of laryngeal function should be carried out using both indirect and direct techniques. The indirect methods include electroglottography (electrolaryngography) and aerodynamic examination. Electroglottography is an electrical impedance method of estimating vocal fold contact during phonation, which is designed to allow investigation of laryngeal microfunction (cycle-by-cycle periodicity and contact).

Aerodynamic measures allow examination of the macrofunctions of the larynx such as laryngeal airflow, glottal pressures and glottal resistance. Estimates of these parameters are obtained by way of the Aerophone II airflow measurement system.

Evaluation of velopharyngeal function

Velopharyngeal function is assessed using a modified version of the nasal accelerometric technique proposed by Horii (1980). The technique involves the use of two miniature accelerometers (Knowles Electronics Model BU-1771), as recommended by Lippmann (1981) to detect nasal and throat vibrations during speech.

Another instrument available for the assessment of nasality is the Nasometer (Kay Elemetrics Model 6200-2). The Nasometer is a computer-assisted instrument that provides a measure of nasality derived from the ratio of acoustic energy output from the nasal and oral cavities during speech.

Evaluation of the articulatory system

The strength, endurance and speed of movement of the muscles of the lips and tongue are assessed by a variety of force transduction systems. A miniaturized pressure transducer (Entran Flatline, Entran Devices Inc., Model EPL-5081-75) with factory calibration, similar to the one described by Hinton and Luschei (1992) can be used to assess lip function. Because of its small size, the transducer is capable of generating interlabial pressure measurements during speech production without interfering with normal articulatory movements.

The tongue force transducer system used by the authors is similar to that described by Robin et al. (1991) and comprises an air-filled soft rubber bulb connected to a pressure transducer. The transducer enables estimation of tongue strength, fine force control and endurance during performance of non-speech tasks only.

Assessment of language

Language assessment needs to be coupled with a comprehensive neuropsychological evaluation and should be an ongoing process in order to monitor possible late effects of treatment (Buttsworth et al., 1993). Depending on the age of the child, a comprehensive assessment would need to examine traditionally considered language areas such as syntax and semantics, as well as literacy and pragmatic skills. It is recommended that the battery include assessments from the *Test of Language Development* (TOLD) series (Hammill and Newcomer, 1982; Newcomer and Hamill, 1982; Hammill et al., 1987) and the *Clinical Evaluation of Language Functions* (CELF) (Semel and Wiig, 1982), supplemented by literacy assessments such as the *Queensland Inventory of Literacy*

(QUIL) and discourse assessments, including the narrative evaluations used by Boon et al. (1994) and Hudson and Murdoch (1992) and other areas of discourse as suggested by Paul (1995). Taylor et al. (1987) used the *Token Test* as part of their assessment battery. Paul (1995) emphasizes the importance of looking at discourse skills from a school or classroom perspective. This is particularly relevant for children following cancer therapy who are attending school, as language for learning is critical in the school-aged child. This approach with children mirrors the examination of functional skills in adults, in a work or social environment.

If word-finding problems are suspected, there are both formal and informal strategies that may be employed to examine these. The *Test of Word Finding* (German, 1986) evaluates students' word-finding skills in constrained naming. German and Simon (1991) also recommend examining children's discourse through elicitation of narratives for language productivity and the incidence of word-finding characteristics. Snyder and Godley (1992) presenta discussion of various formal and informal procedures that may be employed to examine word-finding disorders in children and adolescents.

Treatment of speech and language disorders occurring subsequent to cancer therapy in childhood

Various roles are required of speech/language pathologists in the treatment of the speech and language disorders occurring subsequent to cancer therapy in childhood. Beyond the obvious therapeutic role, an educative role is indicated for speech/language pathologists with the parents, care-givers and teachers of the children. Clinicians must be made aware of the present effects and possible long-term effects of cancer therapy on a child's speech, language, later learning and academic achievement (Buttsworth et al., 1993). In addition to these roles there is the need for the speech/language pathologist to provide ongoing monitoring of the child's speech and language skills.

Treatment of speech disorders

Where developmental speech disorders are identified during the assessment process, either in isolation or in concert with dysarthria, appropriate treatment methodologies must be employed to deal with these disorders.

Developmental disorders

Speech disorders of an articulatory nature have been dealt with in many varied ways by speech/language pathologists. Most traditional approaches emphasize correct placement of articulators and the progression through a hierarchy of tasks beginning with a sound in isolation and ending with transfer into spontaneous speech. Secord (1985) discusses the various traditional approaches to articulation therapy. Whilst the selection of a particular approach to articulation therapy for this population is largely a matter of personal preference, the important factor is the integration of the speech treatment with other aspects of speech and language therapy that the child may require. It is important to bear in mind that certain structures important for motor learning (e.g. the cerebellum) may have been damaged by the cancer or its subsequent treatment. This may occur in children treated for posterior fossa tumours (Murdoch and Hudson-Tennent, 1994). It is not known how this will affect the child's ability to learn the new motor skills, which may be required for the production of speech sounds not present in their repertoire. It may be that more time and emphasis on drill work may be required in therapy in order to learn and establish new speech patterns.

If phonological errors are identified during the assessment process there is a range of approaches that may be employed in therapy. These range from the Metaphon approach as described by Dean et al. (1995), the Cyclic approach as advocated by Hodson and Paden (1991) and various versions of minimal pair therapy. Selection of the appropriate approach must take into consideration other speech difficulties that the child may exhibit and also, importantly the child's language skills, as phonological treatment approaches have a strong language component.

Dysarthria

Current treatment methods for dysarthria in children, particularly for those with acquired dysarthria, are largely modifications of adult methods. This approach has many potential hazards as discussed by Murdoch and Horton (1998), however, the adult treatment methods do provide a starting point from which to proceed in planning and implementing treatment. The strategies discussed below are currently used for the treatment of acquired dysarthria in adults, and have the potential to be used in the child population. Detailed explanations of each approach are provided in Murdoch (1998).

Mutism is frequently reported in the first stages of recovery after brain trauma (Jordan and Murdoch, 1990a, b; Catsman-Berrevoets et al., 1992; Murdoch and Hudson-Tennent, 1994). During this time it is important to provide the child with some form of alternative communication such as a photograph board. After this initial period of mutism the child often presents with severe dysarthria (Catsman-Berrevoets et al., 1992; Murdoch and Hudson-Tennent, 1994). At this time, treatment strategies need to address the goal of improving functional communication and overall intelligibility. Various treatment techniques have been designed to remediate the different functional components of the speech mechanism (i.e. diaphragm, abdomen, rib cage, larynx, velopharynx, tongue, lips and jaw). For patients with speech impairments associated with dysfunction at several different levels of the speech production apparatus, as identified through perceptual and physiological assessment, a treatment framework must be established and the treatment goals prioritized within this framework.

Two treatment frameworks that may be considered are: (a) hierarchical, where each impairment is treated in order of priority; (b) simultaneous, where specific speech impairments, which are interdependent, are treated together.

In many cases it is recommended that the clients receive a treatment programme based on a combination of these methods. Underlying subsystem impairments should be prioritized and treated individually and where appropriate, less system specific impairments can be treated simultaneously. The bases of prioritization for the establishment of the treatment hierarchy are as follows:

1. Severity.
2. Impact on intelligibility.
3. Effect of impairments in a subsystem on other parts of the speech mechanism.

Once the treatment hierarchy has been established the therapeutic approach needs to be determined to aid in selection of specific treatment techniques. There are a number of approaches available to the speech/language pathologist for treating severe dysarthria in children. These include:

- The perceptual approach which uses traditional behavioural techniques (Newman et al., 1985; Rosenbek and LaPointe, 1985; Netsell and Rosenbek, 1986; Crary, 1993).
- The physiological approach which uses instrumental and biofeedback techniques (Netsell and Rosenbek, 1986; Netsell, 1988; Yorkston et al., 1991).
- Prosthetic and surgical techniques (Rosenbek and LaPointe, 1985).
- Augmentative and alternative communication (Murdoch et al., 1990).

In line with the assessment and treatment approaches already mentioned, a combined traditional and physiological treatment approach seems to be indicated in most cases. Of the physiological approaches documented in the literature (Netsell and Rosenbek, 1986) visual biofeedback would seem to be particularly relevant. It provides real-time information regarding the effectiveness of the patient's attempt at a task, an excellent reward system to motivate the subject, and is often simple enough for children to understand and perform on their own (Netsell and Daniel, 1979; Mitchi et al., 1993).

Traditional techniques could also be used, including oro-motor exercises with and without resistance, contrastive stress drills, relaxation and improved posture for respiration (Newman et al., 1985; Rosenbek and LaPointe, 1985; Netsell and Rosenbek, 1986; Crary, 1993).

One approach that seems to have specific relevance to the remediation of the dysarthia of childhood is the PROMPT System (Prompts for Restructuring Oral Muscular Phonetic Targets) devised by Hayden (1994). The system is based on neurological, anatomical and motor theory principles. Using the PROMPT System the phonemic system is translated directly to the neuro-muscular movements required for articulatory sequences. The PROMPT System, uses a tactile basis for guiding the articulatory mechanism and has developed multi-dimensional prompts that may signal various phonemic components such as place, manner, muscle groups and tension of muscle groups, closure, timing and co-articulators influences, during transitive movement, stress and prosodic changes (Hayden and Square, 1994). Hayden has used the system with both children and adults in group and individual settings. She has targeted individuals with disorders including those of phonology, developmental delay, dysarthria, dyspraxia and others. This system coupled with her Motor Speech Treatment Hierarchy (Hayden and Square, 1994) provides a useful additional approach to the assessment and intervention for children and adults with motor speech disorders complementing those mentioned previously.

Treatment of the prosodic disturbances of dysarthria is often more easily carried out in context, using language activities including oral reading (Murdoch et al., 1990). It is, therefore, critical that the speech and language aspects of therapy be closely integrated so that activities may be functional and meaningful. Phrasing, breath group patterning, use of tasks involving volume, stress and intonation can all initially be incorporated into structured language tasks and then gradually into conversational discourse tasks as well.

Treatment of language disorders

Language treatment of a child following cancer therapy, whilst largely directed by the pattern of errors that the child presents with, must have as a key emphasis the development of functional language skills. In particular those language skills required by the child to participate in and succeed at school must be given priority. The ability of school-age children to adjust their messages in light of their listener's needs, to initiate conversation successfully, to ask appropriate questions, to contribute substantively to ongoing conversations, to communicate intentions clearly, to address all participants when joining a group, and to present comments positively more often than negatively have been found to relate to measures of peer acceptance and sociometric status (Gallagher, 1993). The high level of pragmatic functioning required to be a successful communicator whether in the home or at school must be supported by strong skills in the various components of language.

If a child presents with developmental difficulties in the areas of syntax and semantics it is important to deal with these early in the treatment process as these skills are critically important in building the framework for transition into adult grammar and into more literate language development. The goals of intervention, the procedures used and the context for therapy must be considered carefully when designing the intervention programme in order to make it relevant to the child. The characteristics of the child following cancer therapy must be considered to ensure that the programme matches their interest levels as they may be a little older than the children that the clinician usually deals with on these developmental tasks. The clinician should be aware of any other residual effects of cancer therapy that might influence performance (e.g. visual difficulties). Syntax and semantics are hard to separate without making tasks artificial and irrelevant, therefore, they may be worked on in concert using approaches such as whole language, script therapy and activity based intervention (Paul, 1995). Barriers to the child's progression from oral language along the oral–literate continuum to literate language should be identified and dealt with. These include having an age-appropriate vocabulary and good lexical access or word-finding skills.

If word-finding skills have been found to be an area of difficulty for a child it is important to tailor the intervention programme so that the remediation objectives focus on the situational language context that is most difficult for the child. Remediation of word-finding problems in discourse would focus on reducing the presence of word-finding characteristics in the child's narratives. Strategies to be taught would include reflective processing to extinguish repetitions, planning ahead to reduce reformulations and switching to appropriate synonyms to reduce substitutions. Compensatory programming may also need to be considered which involves examining the students strengths and weaknesses and discussing with the school teacher how these could be supported in the classroom. The teacher may need to provide the student with open-ended sentences, descriptions of sentence frames to help cue word retrieval and reduce the amount of unstructured discourse required from the student. Further discussion of strategies for improving memory and word-finding skills may be found in German (1992).

If the child with language difficulties following therapy for cancer is found to have difficulties in the discourse and higher-level language areas, such as using problem-solving strategies and advanced literacy skills, then language therapy needs to occur within the context of school. Initial stages of planning for therapy would need to involve the speech pathologist working closely with the school teacher and parents to plan the programme. Procedures and strategies for modifying the classroom environment and tasks would need to be identified and implemented. The speech pathologist would need to work with the child on the key areas identified using tasks and strategies relevant to the child at school and geared to improving functional outcomes for the child. Paul (1995) has three guiding principles for working with children with difficulties at these levels: first, setting goals that are curriculum-based; second, integrating oral and written language; and third directing conscious attention to the language and cognitive skills the student is using. By using these principles and maintaining a focus on discourse and pragmatic skills the language programme will be functional and relevant to the child's needs.

The most important consideration throughout the whole process of designing the treatment hierarchy, establishing the therapeutic approach and selecting therapy techniques for both speech and language is the need to provide the child with an effective functional communication system. It is important therefore to integrate the speech treatment with the treatment of other communication skills such as language and to use augmentative and alternative communication strategies if necessary.

Case report

The subject, Rebecca, was an 8-year-old female who was admitted to hospital with severe ataxia following a fall down stairs at 6 years of age. A computerized tomography scan upon admission revealed a very large astrocytoma in the posterior cranial fossa. Following stabilization of Rebecca's condition over a period of 6 days, the tumour was removed surgically. After surgery Rebecca spent 5 days in the Intensive Care Unit. On return to the ward little improvement was noted for 4 weeks. A shunt was then inserted with immediate improvement in her condition noted. Daily speech pathology intervention was initiated soon after the initial surgery, with emphasis on decreasing hypersensitivity, reducing gag and bite reflexes and tongue thrust, which were strongly influencing her ability to eat and swallow. One month post-admission Rebecca became a weekly boarder at a specialist centre for children with severe multiple disabilities. Here, she received daily occupational therapy, physiotherapy and speech pathology support. Initially treatment concentrated on feeding skills and oro-motor skills. Three months post-surgery, Rebecca was able to produce some babbling sounds but had difficulty initiating voice. Four months post-surgery Rebecca started talking in single words. Within a fortnight she was using short sentences. Her volume and pitch were poorly controlled and her voice was shaky, with pitch breaks. Rebecca's speech was slow and deliberate and was characterized by the omission of final consonants, reduction of clusters and difficulty with plosives and fricatives. Language comprehension appeared intact in functional situations. Rebecca then made rapid progress in all areas. She demonstrated some perseveration in conversation and had difficulty changing topics and activities. Rebecca continued in the intensive placement for another 4 months. Rebecca returned home 8 months post-surgery and was supported with weekly visits in her local school by a regional therapy team for several months. Speech pathology services were then suspended for a period of 9 months. After this break Rebecca received bimonthly visits from the regional speech pathologist to review her speech and language skills. At 30 months post-surgery, Rebecca began receiving weekly speech pathology intervention concentrating on developing her higher-level expressive language, reasoning and narrative skills. At this time, her speech was reported to be intelligible with a slow rate, and even and equal stress patterns. When prompted, Rebecca was able to modulate stress for expression and emphasis during story telling.

Neuropsychological assessment carried out 23 months post-surgery indicated that Rebecca's general level of cognitive functioning at that time was within the borderline range. However, her overall performance on verbal comprehension tests was significantly higher than her overall performance on visuoperceptual tests. She had some short-term memory problems and had particular difficulty with memory for visual material. Rebecca's visuospatial skills were severely impaired as were visuomotor speed and visual scanning. Basic verbal fluency, higher-level verbal expression and verbal comprehension were within the average range.

At 27 months post-surgery Rebecca was referred for a comprehensive perceptual and physiological analysis of her speech.

Perceptual analysis of speech

Rebecca was given the same battery of perceptual assessments as described in the Assessment section above. The perceptual assessment indicated that Rebecca had a mild dysarthric speech impairment mainly characterized by the use of a slow rate of speech. Even though there was some impairment to tongue and lip movements Rebecca's speech was intelligible. No developmental speech errors were noted.

Physiological analysis of speech

A detailed report of the findings of the physiological analysis of Rebecca's speech is presented in Chapter 8. A brief report of the physiological findings is outlined below.

Respiratory function, as assessed through clinical spirometry showed, Rebecca to have lung volumes and capacities well below the predicted values for her age, sex and height. This finding is in contrast to that reported for a group of children with dysarthria resulting from treatment for posterior fossa tumours reported by Murdoch and Hudson-Tennent (1994). Rebecca also performed differently to the group reported above in that she showed consistently high abdominal and rib cage termination values across all tasks, resulting in high lung volume termination values. For syllable and reading tasks, Rebecca's inspiratory volumes were generally lower than expected, resulting in an overall reduction in chest wall excursion and leading to lower lung excursion and poorer breath support for speech. Calculation of relative volume contribution showed Rebecca to be a predominantly abdominal breather.

Instrumental investigation of laryngeal and velopharyngeal function indicated Rebecca's skills to be within normal limits.

Although Rebecca had tongue pressure and endurance levels that were within normal limits, she produced a significantly reduced number of repetitions on a timed task. It could be hypothesized that Rebecca reduced the number of repetitions in order to preserve the strength and accuracy of the movements. This would be in keeping with the perceptual observation of reduced rate of speech and maintenance of intelligibility. The lip pressure transducer analysis indicated that Rebecca's maximum lip pressure on non-speech tasks was reduced as was her lip pressure during bilabial consonant production in speech. However, this did not appear to lead to noticeable bilabial consonant distortions as this was not noted to be deviant in the perceptual assessment.

Implications for treatment — speech

Rebecca presented with a mild dysarthria characterized by prosodic changes detected by the perceptual assessment. Physiological assessment revealed respiratory and articulatory system difficulties, which although not detected perceptually, may well have contributed to the major area of concern (i.e. reduced rate of speech). It may be hypothesized that Rebecca was reducing her speech rate in order to conserve expiratory output and ensure accuracy and strength of articulatory movements. Treatment would, therefore, concentrate on the following areas:

1. Treatment of prosodic aspects of speech, particularly rate and intonation:
   Increase speech rate
   Improve use of intonation patterns
2. Treatment of respiratory dysfunction:
   Increase lung volumes and capacities
   Decrease abdominal and rib cage termination volumes during speech
3. Treatment of articulatory dysfunction:
   Increase lip strength
   Increase tongue strength.

Owing to the nature of the systems requiring treatment and their inter-relatedness the recommended treatment framework would be more simultaneous rather than hierarchical. It is believed in this case that the treatment of prosodic dysfunction will enhance Rebecca's communication skills. Treatment techniques for prosody could include the use of breath group patterning in concert with treatment for respiratory–phonatory control to enable Rebecca to produce longer breath groups. The use of reading and drama-based activities could be successful as Rebecca was able to read short passages 'with expression'.

Implications for treatment — language

Although Rebecca's language skills were not reassessed at the time of speech assessment, treatment priorities could be generated from earlier reports and from discussion with her speech pathologist, teacher and family. The main areas of language difficulty were occurring in the classroom where Rebecca was having difficulty processing verbal information at a rapid rate. Speech pathology intervention would focus on working with the classroom teacher to modify her approach to providing information to Rebecca to allow for her increased processing time. Rebecca would need to be taught strategies for managing information and improving her problem-solving skills to ensure that she maximized her information-processing skills. A regular assessment cycle would be built into the periods of therapy and review in order to monitor Rebecca's language skills on an ongoing basis and to ensure that she was coping with the pace and the demands of the classroom.

Conclusions

Although the presence and nature of speech and language disturbances following cancer therapy in childhood are variable, the information presented above points to a key role for the speech/language pathologist in the management of these children. This role can involve the monitoring of a child's communication skills. In some cases the speech/language pathologist will also need to implement an intensive therapeutic programme involving the treatment of both speech and language disabilities. These roles must be supported by ongoing research into the nature and course of speech and language disorders in children following treatment for cancer.

References

Boon DL, Murdoch BE, Jordan FM (1994) Performance on creative narrative tasks of children treated for acute lymphocytic leukaemia. Aphasiology 8: 549–568.

Boren HG, Kory RC, Syner JC (1966) The Veterans Administration Army cooperative study of pulmonary function II: The lung volume and its subdivisions in normal men. American Journal of Medicine 41: 96–114.

Broadbent VA, Barnes ND, Wheeler TK (1981) Medulloblastoma in childhood: long-term results of treatment. Cancer 48: 26–30.

Brouwers P, Riccardi R, Fedio P, Poplack DG (1985) Long-term neuropsychologic sequelae of childhood leukemia: correlation with CT brain scan abnormalities.

Journal of Pediatrics 106: 723–728.

Buttsworth DL, Murdoch BE, Ozanne AE (1993) Acute lymphoblastic leukaemia: language deficits in children post-treatment. Disability and Rehabilitation 15: 67–75.

Carrow-Woolfolk E, Lynch J (1982) An Integrated Approach to Language Disorders in Children. Orlando, FL: Grune & Stratton.

Catsman-Berrevoets CE, Van Dongen HR, Zwetsloot CP (1992) Transient loss of speech followed by dysarthria after removal of posterior fossa tumour. Developmental Medicine and Child Neurology 34: 1102–1117.

Copeland DR, Fletcher JM, Pfefferbaum-Levine B, Jaffe N, Reid H, Maor N (1985) Neuropsychological sequelae of childhood cancer in long-term survivors. Pediatrics 75: 745–753.

Crary MA (1993) Developmental Motor Speech Disorders. San Diego, CA: Singular Publishing Group.

Danoff BF, Chowchock FS, Marquette C, Mulgrew L, Kramer S (1982) Assessment of the long-term effects of primary radiation therapy for brain tumours in children. Cancer 49: 1580–1586.

Darley FL, Aronson AE, Brown JR (1975) Motor Speech Disorders. Philadelphia, PA: WB Saunders.

Dean EC, Howell J, Waters D, Reid J (1995) Metaphon: a metalinguistic approach to the treatment of phonological disorder in children. Clinical Linguistics and Phonetics 9: 1–19.

Eiser C (1978) Intellectual abilities among survivors of childhood leukaemia as function of CNS irradiation. Archives of Disease in Childhood 53: 391–395.

Eiser C (1980) Effects of chronic illness on intellectual development: a comparison of normal children with those treated for childhood leukaemia and solid tumours. Archives of Disease in Childhood 55: 766–770.

Enderby P (1983) Frenchay Dysarthria Assessment. San Diego, CA: College-Hill Press.

Fisher HB, Logemann JA (1971) The Fisher–Logemann Test of Articulation Competence. Boston, MA: Houghton Mifflin.

FitzGerald FJ, Murdoch BE, Chenery HJ (1987) Multiple sclerosis: associated speech and language disorders. Australian Journal of Communication Disorders 15: 15–35.

Gallagher TM (1993) Language skill and the development of social competence in school-age children. Language, Speech, and Hearing Services in Schools 24: 199–205.

Garcia-Perez A, Sierrasesumaga L, Narbona-Garcia J, Calvo-Manual F, Aguirre-Ventallo M (1994) Neuropsychological evaluation of children with intracranial tumours: impact of treatment modalities. Medical and Pediatric Oncology 23: 116–123.

German DJ (1986) National College of Education, Test of Word Finding (TWF). Allen, TX: DLM Teaching Resources.

German DJ (1992) Word-finding intervention for children and adolescents. Topics in Language Disorders 13: 33–50.

German DJ, Simon E (1991) Analysis of children's word-finding skills in discourse. Journal of Speech and Hearing Research 34: 309–316.

Hammill DD, Newcomer PL (1982) Test of Language Development — Intermediate. Austin, TX: Pro-Ed.

Hammill DD, Brown VL, Larsen SC, Wiederhold JL (1987) Test of Adolescent Language 2: A Multidimensional Approach to Assessment. Austin, TX: Pro-Ed.

Hayden DA (1994) The P.R.O.M.P.T. System. Extended Level 1: Certification Manual (revised edition). Toronto, Ontario: The PROMPT Institute.

Hayden DA, Square PA (1994) Motor speech treatment hierarchy: a systems approach. Clinics in Communication Disorders 4: 162–174.

Hinton VA, Luschei ES (1992) Validation of a modern miniature transducer for measurement of interlabial contact pressure during speech. Journal of Speech and Hearing Research, 35, 245–251.

Hodson B, Paden E (1991) Targeting Intelligible Speech: A Phonological Approach to Remediation. San Diego, CA: College-Hill Press.

Horii Y (1980) An accelerometric approach to nasality measurement: a preliminary report. Cleft Palate Journal 17: 254–261.

Hudson LJ, Murdoch BE (1992) Chronic language deficits in children treated for posterior fossa tumours. Aphasiology 6: 135–150.

Hudson LJ, Murdoch BE, Ozanne AE (1989) Posterior fossa tumours in childhood: associated speech and language disorders post-surgery. Aphasiology 3: 1–18.

Jackel CA, Murdoch BE, Ozanne AE, Buttsworth DL (1990) Language abilities of children treated for acute lymphoblastic leukaemia: preliminary findings. Aphasiology 4: 45–53.

Jenney MEM, Kane RL, Lurie N (1995) Developing a measure of health outcomes in survivors of childhood cancer: a review of the issues. Medical and Pediatric Oncology 24:145–153.

Johnston JR (1982) Narratives: a new look at communication problems in older language-disordered children. Language, Speech and Hearing Services in Schools 13: 144–155.

Jordan FM, Murdoch BE (1990a) Linguistic status following closed head injury in children: a follow-up study. Brain Injury 4: 147–154.

Jordan FM, Murdoch BE (1990b) Unexpected recovery of functional communication following a prolonged period of mutism post-head injury. Brain Injury 4: 101–108.

Koh PS, Raffensperger JG, Berry S, Larsen MB, Johnstone HS, Chou P, Luck SR, Hammer M, Cohn SL (1994) Long-term outcome in children with opsoclonus-myoclonus and ataxia and coincident neuroblastoma. Journal of Pediatrics 125: 712–716.

Kory RC, Callahan R, Boren HG (1961) The Veterans Administration Army cooperative study of pulmonary function I: Clinical spirometry in normal men. American Journal of Medicine 30: 243–258.

Lippmann RP (1981) Detecting nasalisation using a low cost miniature accelerometer. Journal of Speech and Hearing Research 24: 314–317.

Michi K, Yamashita Y, Imai S, Suzuki N, Yoshida H et al. (1993) Role of visual feedback treatment for defective /s/ sounds in patients with cleft palate. Journal of Speech and Hearing Research 36: 277–285.

Murdoch BE (1998) Dysarthria. A Physiological Approach to Assessment and Treatment. Cheltenham: Stanley Thornes.

Murdoch BE, Horton SK (1998) Acquired and developmental dysarthria in childhood. In Murdoch BE (ed.) Dysarthria. A Physiological Approach to Assessment and Treatment. Cheltenham: Stanley Thornes: 373–427.

Murdoch BE, Hudson-Tennent LJ (1994) Differential language outcomes in children following treatment for posterior fossa tumours. Aphasiology 8: 507–534.

Murdoch B, Chenery H, Bowler S, Ingram J (1989) Respiratory function in Parkinson's subjects exhibiting a perceptible speech deficit: a kinematic and spirometric analysis. Journal of Speech and Hearing Disorders 54: 610–626.

Murdoch BE, Ozanne AE, Cross JA (1990) Acquired childhood speech disorders: dysarthria and dyspraxia. In Murdoch BE (Ed.) Acquired Neurological Speech/Language Disorders in Childhood. London: Taylor & Francis, 308–341.

Murdoch BE, Boon DL, Ozanne AE (1994) Variability of language outcomes in children treated for acute lymphoblastic leukaemia: an examination of 23 cases. Journal of Medical Speech/Language Pathology 2: 113–123.

Netsell R (1988) Physiological studies of dysarthria and their relevance to treatment. Seminars in Speech and Language 5: 279–291.

Netsell R, Daniel B (1979) Dysarthria in adults: physiologic approach in rehabilitation. Archives of Physical Medicine and Rehabilitation 60: 502–508.

Netsell R, Lotz WK, Barlow SM (1989) A speech physiology examination for individuals with dysarthria. In Yorkston KM, Beukelman DR (eds) Recent Advances in Clinical Dysarthria. Boston, MA: College-Hill Press, 4–37.

Netsell R, Rosenbek J (1986) Treating the dysarthrias. In Netsell R (Ed.) A Neurobiologic View of Speech Production and the Dysarthrias. San Diego, CA: College-Hill Press, 123–152.

Newcomer PL, Hammill DD (1982) Test of Language Development-Primary. Austin, TX: Pro-Ed.

Newman PW, Creaghead NA, Secord W (1985) Assessment and Remediation of Articulatory and Phonological Disorders. Columbus, OH: Charles E Merrill.

Pantell RH, Lewis CC (1987) Measuring the impact of medical care on children. Journal of Chronic Disease 40 (Suppl 1): 99s–108s.

Paul R (1995) Language Disorders from Infancy through Adolescence. Assessment and Intervention. St Louis: Mosby.

Rekate HL, Grubb RL, Aram DM, Hahn JF, Ratcheson RA (1985) Muteness of cerebellar origin. Archives of Neurology 42: 697–698.

Robin DA, Somodi LB, Luschei ES (1991) Measurement of strength and endurance in normal and articulation disordered subjects. In Moore CA, Yorkston KM, Beukelman, DR (eds) Dysarthria and Apraxia of Speech: perspectives on management. Baltimore, MD: Paul H Brooks, 173–184.

Rosenbek JC, La Pointe LL (1985) The dysarthrias: description, diagnosis, and treatment. In Johns D (Ed.) Clinical Management of Neurogenic Communication Disorders. Boston, MA: Little, Brown & Co, 97–152.

Secord W (1985) The traditional approach to articulation treatment. In Newman PW, Creaghead NA, Secord W (eds) Assessment and Remediation of Articulatory and Phonological Disorders. Columbus, OH: Charles E Merrill, 127–158.

Semel EM, Wiig EH (1982) Clinical Evaluation of Language Functions. Columbus, OH: Charles E Merrill.

Snyder LS, Godley D (1992) Assessment of word-finding disorders in children and adolescents. Topics in Language Disorders 13: 15–32.

Taylor HG, Albo VC, Phebus CK, Sachs BR, Bierl PG (1987) Postirradiation treatment outcomes for children with acute lymphocytic leukaemia: clarification of risks. Journal of Pediatric Psychology 12: 395–411.

Volcan I, Cole GP, Johnston K (1986) A case of muteness of cerebellar origin. Archives of Neurology 43: 313–314.

Yorkston J, Beukelman D (1981) Assessment of Intelligibility of Dysarthric Speech. Austin, TX: Pro-Ed.

Yorkston KM, Beukelman DR, Bell KR (1991) Clinical Management of Dysarthric Speakers. Philadelphia, PA: Taylor & Francis.

Index